THE OFFICIAL FIVE STAR FITNESS

BOOT CAMP
WORKOUT

UPDATED EDITION

FOR MEN AND WOMEN

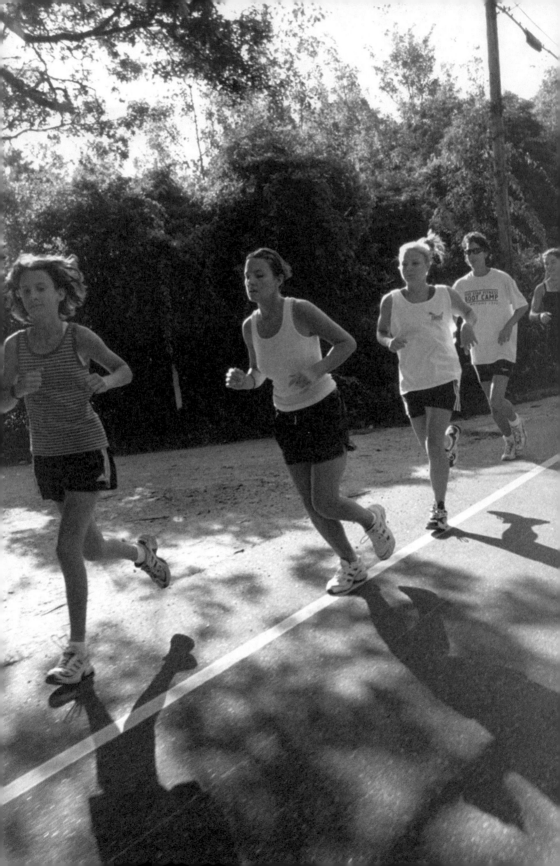

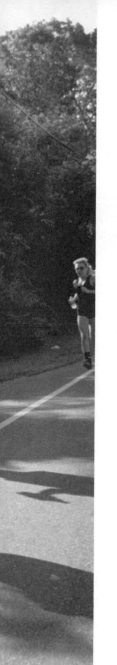

THE OFFICIAL FIVE STAR FITNESS

BOOT CAMP WORKOUT

UPDATED EDITION
FOR MEN AND WOMEN

WRITTEN BY
Andrew Flach, Paul Frediani
and Stew Smith

PHOTOGRAPHY
Peter Field Peck

Hatherleigh/Five Star Fitness
New York

Hatherleigh Press
5-22 46th Ave, Suite 200
Long Island City, NY 11101
1-800-528-2550
www.getfitnow.com

Library of Congress Cataloging-in-Publication Data

Flach, Andrew, 1961-
  The official five star fitness boot camp workout / written by Andrew
Flach, Paul Frediani and Stew Smith ; photography by Peter Field Peck. --
Updated ed.
      p. cm.
  ISBN 978-1-57826-243-4
  1. Exercise. 2. Physical fitness. I. Frediani, Paul, 1952- II. Smith,
Stewart, 1969- III. Title.
  GV481.F5513 2007
  613.7--dc22
                                            2007010716

Before beginning any strenuous exercise program, consult your physician. The authors and publisher of this book and workout disclaim any liability, person or professional, resulting from the misapplication of any of the training procedures described in this publication.

All Five Star Fitness titles are available for schools, bulk purchase, special promotions, and premiums. For more information, please contact the manager of our Marketing and Sales Department at 1-800-528-2550.

Cover design by Lisa Fyfe

Text design and composition by Elina Nudelman

Photographed by Peter Field Peck

Military vehicles courtesy of Andrew Flach

Printed in the United States
10 9 8 7 6 5 4 3 2

Acknowledgments

The authors are grateful to the following persons for their contributions to the success of the Boot Camp:

Don Eames, Post Commander, and Ralph James, American Legion East Hampton Post for use of the American Legion Hall facilities

Jill Gilbert, a personal trainer and our beautiful fitness model who appears throughout the book

Beth Simpson and Claudine Setera of Polar Products for use of their equipment

Bill Bishop of SoBe Beverages for quenching our parched thirsts

Pete "Pistol" Gilman of Soffe who dressed us for success

Al Shelton, our landlord, for putting us up (or was it putting up with us?)

Trish and Fred Mittman, for his skill and tools and her good cooking

Gabrielle Costanzo of Beach Radio, and her father Conrad, for their boundless enthusiasm

Matt Bloom, a great friend who skillfully drove "Drake" (our M35A2 cargo truck!) from Chicago to NY

Bruce Slagle, Imran Masood, and all the other members of the Five Star Fitness Team

Lisa Fyfe and Elina Nudelman, our excellent designers

Tracy Tumminello, our in-house wordsmith, whose talent shines on every page

Finally, and most importantly,

Those of you who showed up for class...thank you!

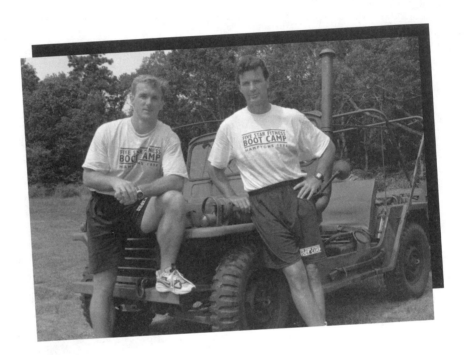

Welcome Fitness Recruits!

The Five Star Fitness team has assembled the most complete, instructive, and challenging workout that requires little or no major exercise equipment. The Five Star Fitness Boot Camp Workout is modeled after the workout programs of the most fit military units in the world: The United States Navy, Air Force, Army, and Marine Corps!

Now, this does not mean that YOU cannot excel at this workout program. We have designed this program to change anyone from a sedentary beginner to a "lean, mean, fit machine." Do not be concerned with the terminology at Five Star Fitness. Your Five Star Fitness instructors, as well as the United States Armed Forces, feel the term "BOOT CAMP" means "BEGINNING." This is a beginning fitness program for those who need the motivation of the Armed Forces to start and continue a lifestyle of fitness. We will help you reach your goals IF you stay motivated like the men and women who protect and serve this country for all of us. *So, there is no need to be intimidated by this workout program*—ANYBODY CAN DO IT!

The Five Star Fitness Boot Camp Workout concentrates on building lean muscle mass through calisthenics and weight training, and by burning fat through aerobic exercise. Contrary to some beliefs, there is no magic pill to losing weight and being fit. You have to eat right and exercise. Your Five Star Fitness instructors will demonstrate how to do both.

SO—ATTENTION! TIME TO EXERCISE!

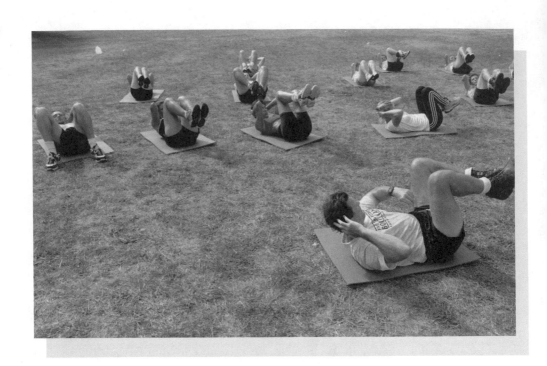

Contents

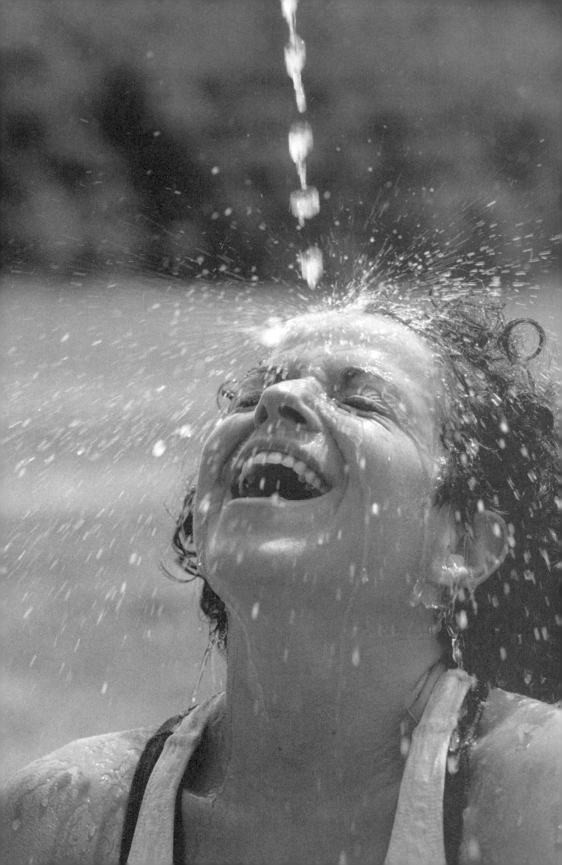

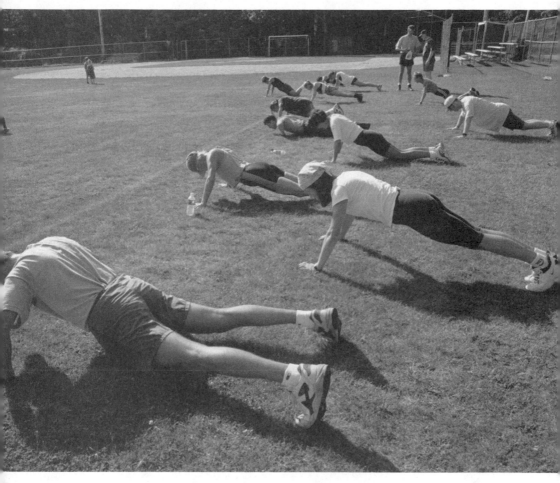

Part I

Introduction

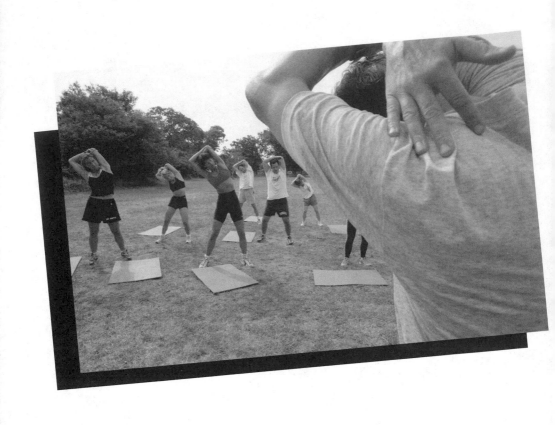

Introd

Introduction

Thanks for picking up this copy of the Official Five Star Fitness Boot Camp Workout. Something about it must have caught your attention. Perhaps it was the phrase "Boot Camp," which suggests a military-style fitness program. Maybe it was the great photos of people having fun with fitness (and fitness should be fun!). Whatever the reason, in these pages you will find the most dynamic and diverse fitness program ever presented.

The idea for the book came to me while I was researching several books on fitness and physical training in the United States Armed Forces. To date, we have published five books on military exercise programs and have documented the training regimens of the United States Navy SEALs, Air Force PJ's and CCT's, Marine Corps, and Naval Academy. For the background work on these books, we visited training bases around the country where we witnessed first hand the rigorous calisthenics-based programs of the military service branches.

As we watched from the sidelines, it was hard to resist the desire to join the training sessions. There was a unique motivational energy involved with outdoor group training *en masse*. It was exciting to witness the simple yet profound sequence of exercises. They required little to no equipment and could be done anywhere. This was a refreshing sight considering the modern trend towards expensive health clubs with complex technological fitness machinery.

And so I thought, 'wouldn't it be great to bring this to life for civilians'—back-to-basics fitness! These were the kinds of exercises we hated to do in high school gym class, but now were eager to try again—jumping jacks, push-ups, pull-ups, all done in the fresh open air!

After a month-long search, we were fortunate enough to enlist the cooperation of the American Legion East Hampton Post, which allowed us to use their field every Saturday and Sunday throughout July and August of 1998. We built pull-up bars and a platform for the exercise instructor. We acquired more than a thousand pounds of dumbbells and a couple of dozen ammo cans (to fill with sand for challenging lunges). We bought a case of bananas and four watermelons. We were ready!

The first weekend of operation was a near disaster! Although we had great weather, almost no one showed up. But, over the next few weekends, word spread and we were rewarded with a steady stream of men and women interested in our innovative approach to fitness. We were also blessed with fantastic weather.

By the end of the summer, we were sad to say goodbye to Boot Camp, but fortunately we thoroughly documented our training program for year-round results! And so we offer this book to you as our way of encouraging you to get fit and stay fit throughout your life.

And remember, when it comes to fitness, there's no excuse not to do something!

Andrew Flach

Many people recognize the need to make exercise an integral part of their lives, however they don't know where to start. They ask themselves:

- Where will I exercise?

- How much will it cost?

- How often do I have to exercise?

- Do I have time to exercise?

- How do I exercise safely?

You can exercise in the convenience of your own home with the help of this book, or you can buy a gym membership. Gym memberships usually cost anywhere from $30 to $100 a month, with most of all of that money paid up front for the three to six month membership.

It is best to exercise at least five times a week. Your workout sessions can be as short as 20 to 30 minutes in length. The bottom line is that you HAVE to take time out of your schedule for fitness. You make time for work, studies, family, daily errands, daily or weekly worship; you have to make time for your health as well. Your health HAS to be a priority in your life.

Any book in the Five Star Fitness Series will show you the way to exercise in an inexpensive, safe, and highly effective manner.

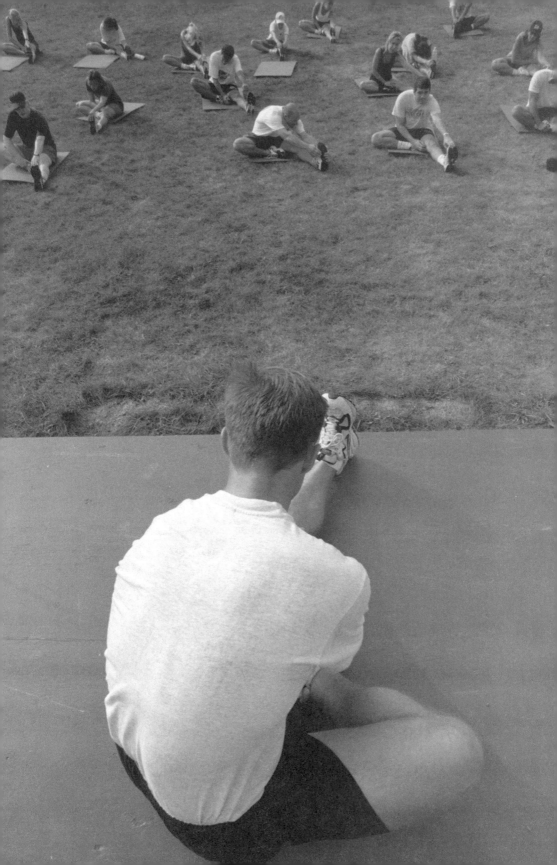

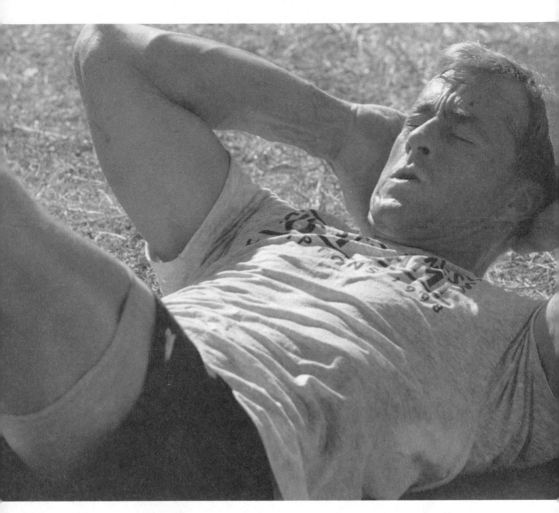

The Exercises

Stretching & Flexibility

Flexibility exercises, more commonly referred to as *stretching*, are vital to any physical fitness conditioning program. There are numerous benefits to beginning a stretching program. Stretching makes the joints and muscles more pliable and less susceptible to everyday injuries, helps relieve everyday stress, and reduces muscle soreness after exercising. In fact, Five Star Fitness instructors strongly encourage beginners who have not exercised in years to devote a full week to stretching prior to beginning an exercise program. If you're a beginner, you will be glad you did. Once you are more flexible and ready to begin an exercise program, Five Star Fitness instructors will have you complete a flexibility routine before and after every workout.

Before you stretch, you must warm up your muscles. Take a quarter mile jog or do an easy calisthenic exercise, such as twenty-five jumping jacks. It is absolutely crucial to warm-up before any type of workout. A warm-up increases both the temperature of your muscles and your heart rate, in turn preparing your body for the increased stress of physical exercise. When you properly prepare your muscles, tendons, ligaments and heart for a workout, exercise is more efficient and safer.

& Flexibility

Things to keep in mind while performing the flexibility exercises:

- Stretch to the point of tightness and hold that position for 15 seconds before you workout. Hold each stretch for 30 seconds after you workout.

- Do not bounce when stretching. Bouncing initiates the stretch reflex, causing muscles to tighten rather than relax. It also increases the chance of injury to muscles and joints.

Your Pre-Training "Stretch Week"

Schedule: First seven days (30 seconds each stretch).

Neck Stretch	Hip Rotations
Arm / Shoulder Stretch	Thigh Stretch
Arm Circles	Hamstring Stretch
Tricep / Back Stretch	Inner Thigh Side Stretch
Chest Stretch	Hurdler Stretch
Shoulder Rotations	ITB (iliotibial band) Stretch
Cobra Ab Stretch	Butterfly Stretch
Knees to Chest	Calf / Achilles Tendon Stretch

*After the first week, the "stretch week" schedule becomes your pre-workout routine.

The Stretches

NECK

Turn your head to the left, right, up and down, as if you were nodding "yes" and "no." Do this stretch slowly. You do not want to raise, lower, or rotate your neck too much. You can cause neck injury if you do not perform this stretch in a slow and relaxing fashion.

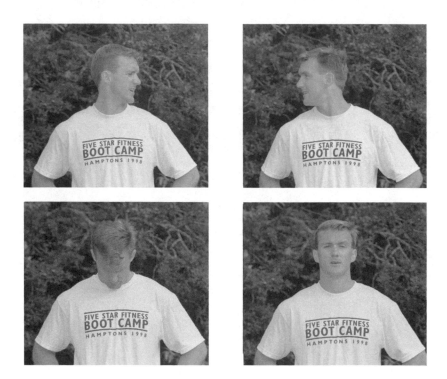

This stretch is a great tension reliever in the base of your neck. While you are sitting down at the office, the neck stretch can help you prevent or eliminate tension headaches.

ARM / SHOULDER

Drop your shoulder and pull your arm across your chest. With the opposite arm, gently pull your arm across your chest and hold for 15 seconds. Repeat with the other arm.

This exercise will stretch the back of the shoulder and muscles that attach the shoulder blade to the upper part of the back. This is the very root of most tension headaches.

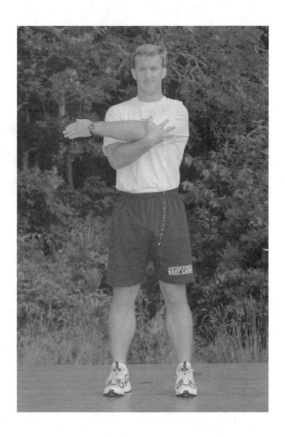

ARM CIRCLES

Rotate your arms slowly in big circles forward and reverse for 15 seconds in each direction. This will prepare your shoulders for such exercises as push-ups, dips, and dumbbell work.

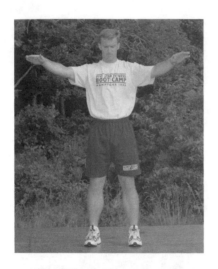
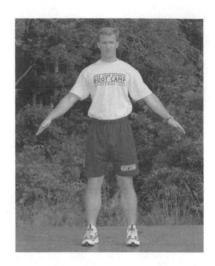
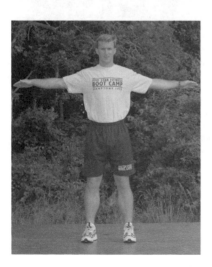
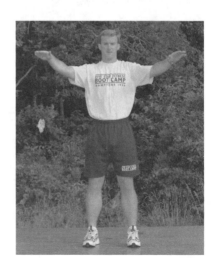

CHEST

Stand with your arms extended and parallel to the floor. Slowly pull your elbows back as far as you can. Hold for 15 seconds. Do not thrust your arms backwards. This is a slow and deliberate stretch designed to prepare your chest for push-ups, dips, and other shoulder/chest exercises.

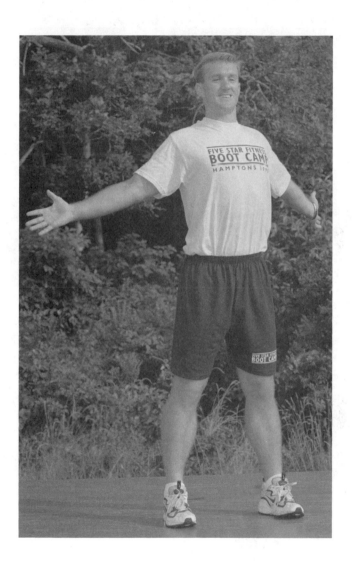

TRICEPS INTO BACK STRETCH

Place both arms over and behind your head. Grab your right elbow with your left hand and pull your elbow toward your opposite shoulder. Lean with the pull. Repeat with the other arm.

This stretch not only prepares you for the dumbbell triceps exercises, push-ups, and dips, but also prepares the back muscles for pull-ups! This is a very important stretch for upper body exercises!

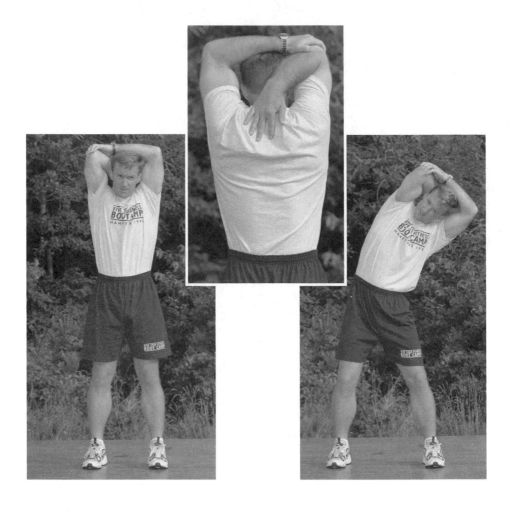

SHOULDER ROTATIONS

Rotate your shoulders slowly up and down, keeping your arms relaxed by your side. Your shoulders should rotate in small circles and move up and down in slow distinct movements.

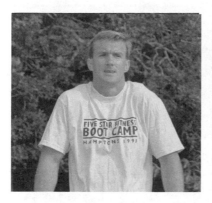 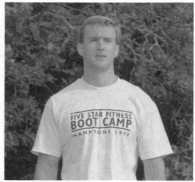

FOREARM STRETCH

When you are cranking out myriad pull-up combinations and pyramids, your forearms might start to get tight (or numb). One way to ease the discomfort is by regularly stretching between sets.

To perform this stretch, reach one arm out front with your palm flat and face up. Reach over with your free hand and gently grab across your fingers. Press down and back, feeling the stretch in your forearm. For variation, hold your palm face down and press up and back with your free hand. As in all stretches, you should feel slight discomfort, but not pain. If you feel pain, discontinue the exercise.

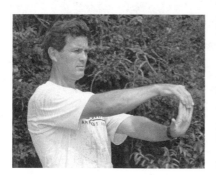 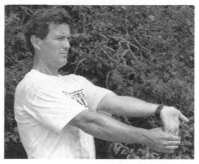

COBRA AB STRETCH

Lay on your stomach and push yourself up on your elbows. Slowly lift your head and shoulders and look up at the sky or ceiling. Hold for 15 seconds and repeat two times.

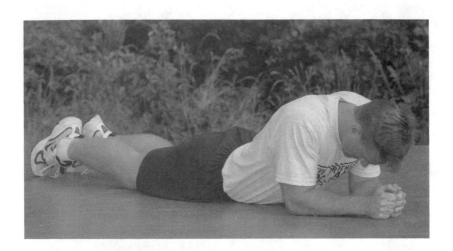

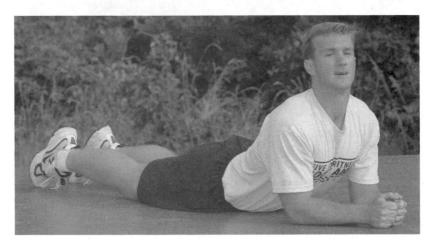

KNEES TO CHEST

Lay flat on your back. Pull your knees to your stomach and hold for 20 seconds. You should perform this stretch before and after any abdominal exercise.

As you may know, the lower back is the most commonly injured area of the body.

Many lower back problems stem from inactivity, lack of flexibility, and the improper lifting of heavy objects. Stretching and exercising your lower back will help prevent some of those injuries.

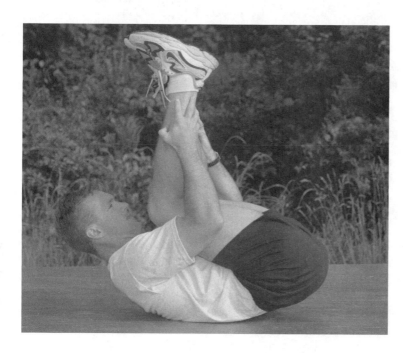

HIP ROTATIONS

Place your hands on your hips and slowly rotate your hips in big circles clockwise and counterclockwise for about 15 seconds in each direction.

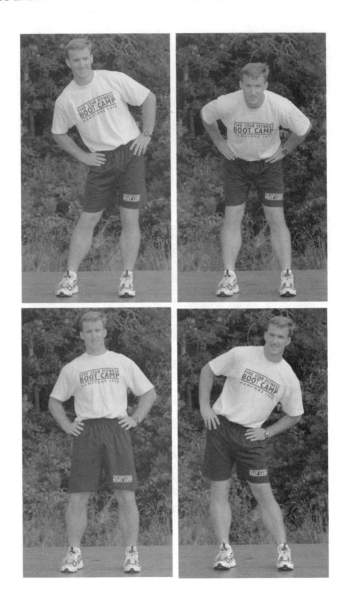

THIGH STRETCH STANDING

Standing, bend your knee and grab your foot at the ankle. Pull your heel to your butt, keeping your knees close together. Hold for 10 to 15 seconds and repeat with the other leg. (You can hold onto something for balance if you need to OR you can pull on your opposite ear - somehow this helps you keep your balance!)

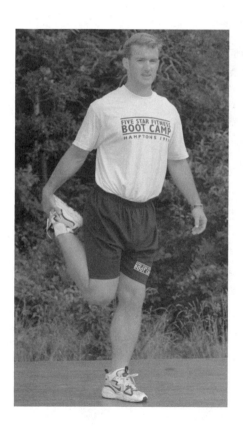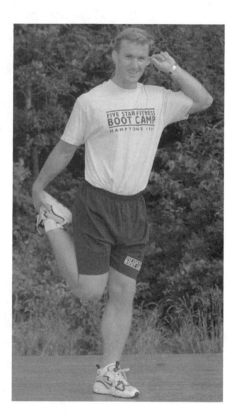

HAMSTRING STRETCH

From the standing or sitting position, bend forward at the waist and touch your toes. Keep your back straight and slightly bend your knees. You should feel this stretching the back of your thighs.

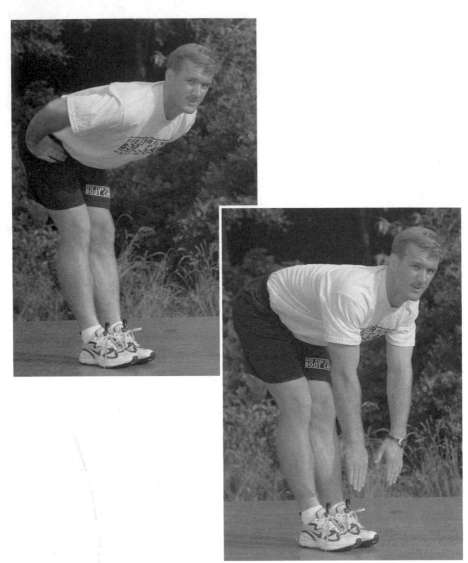

INNER THIGH SIDE STRETCH

Stand with your legs spread and lean to the left/right. Keep the foot of the straightened leg pointing toes up.

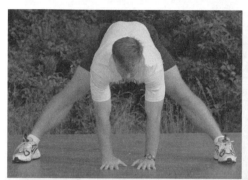
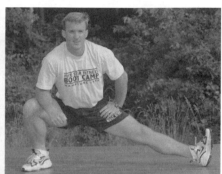

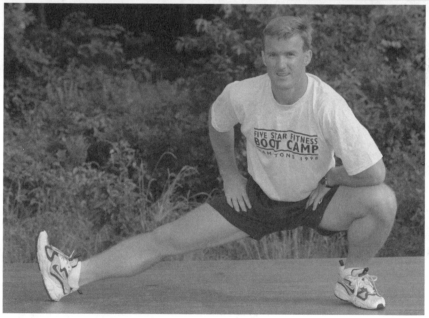

THIGH STRETCH ON GROUND

Lie down on your left side. Pull your right foot to your butt by grabbing your ankle and holding it with your right hand. Keep your knees close together and hold for 10 to 15 seconds. Repeat with the other leg.

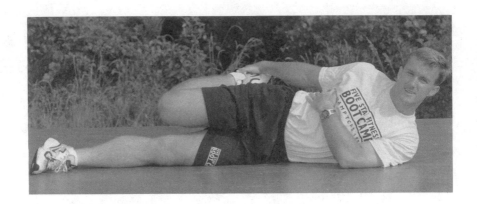

HURDLER STRETCH

Sit on the floor with your legs straight in front of you. Bend your right knee and place the bottom of your foot on the inside of your opposite thigh. With your back straight, lean forward to stretch the back of your legs and your lower back. Hold the stretch for 15 seconds, switch legs and repeat.

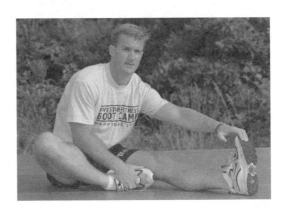

ITB (ILIOTIBIAL BAND) STRETCH

Sit on the ground with your legs crossed in front of you. Keeping your legs crossed, bring the top leg to your chest and bend it at the knee so that your foot is placed outside your opposite leg's thigh. Hold your knee for 15 seconds against your chest and repeat with the other leg.

You should perform this stretch before and after running. This will help prevent common overuse injuries in the hips and knees.

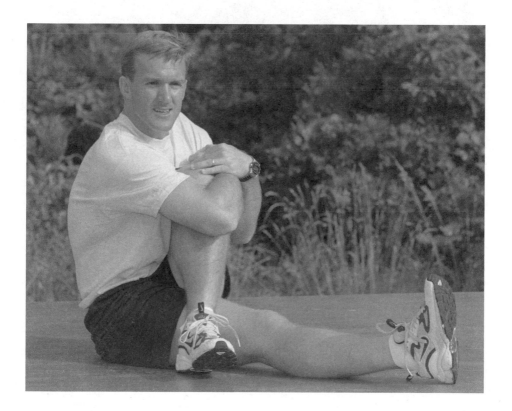

BUTTERFLY

Sit upright with your knees bent and the soles of your feet together. Grab your ankles and place both of your elbows on your inner thighs. Slowly push down on your thighs. This stretch helps to loosen the groin and inner thighs.

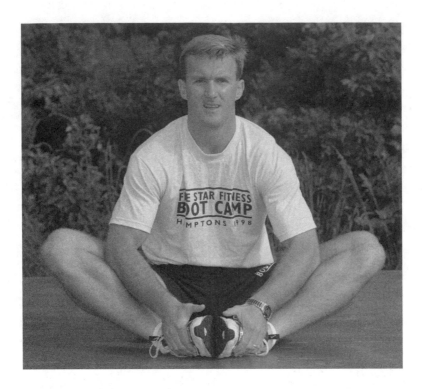

CALF STRETCH INTO ACHILLES TENDON STRETCH

Stand with one foot two to three feet in front of the other. With both feet pointing in the same direction as you are facing. Put most of your body weight on the leg that is behind you, stretching the calf muscle.

Now, bend the rear knee slightly. You should now feel the stretch in your heel. This stretch helps prevent Achilles tendonitis, a severe injury that will sideline most people for about four to six weeks.

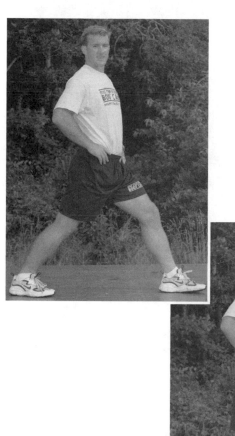

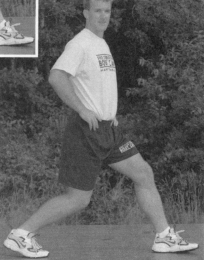

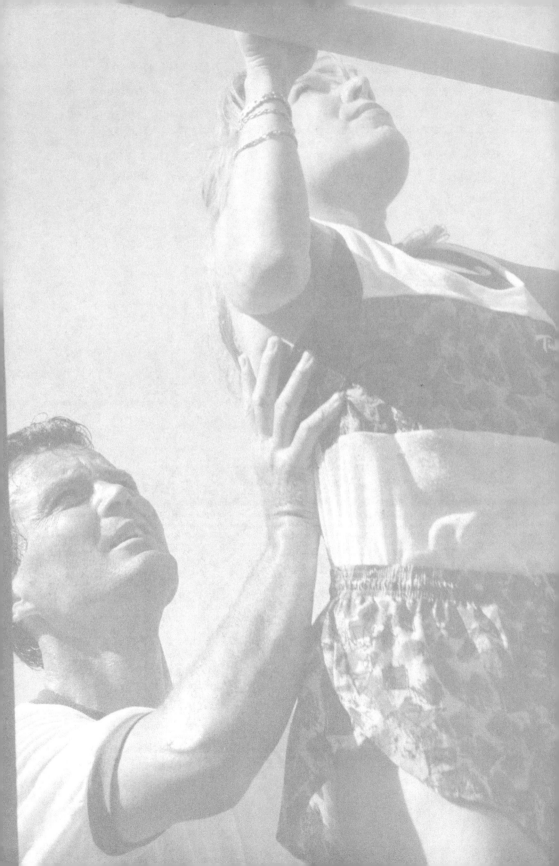

Upper Body
Calisthenic Exercises

Push-ups are the all-time favorite exercise of the military and with good reason. This is an effective exercise that helps build the shoulders, chest, and arms, and strengthens the core, abdominal, and lower-back muscles. You will be performing several different types of push-ups, each working a different part of the chest, arms, and shoulders.

In the not-so-distant past, many people felt pull-ups and regular push-ups were a gender specific exercise, meaning only men could perform these exercises. This perception, of course, is a myth. In fact, there are many men who cannot perform any pull-ups and push-ups and many women who can. The common denominator between the men and women who can perform these upper body exercises is: They practice pull-ups and push-ups.

PUSH-UP

REGULAR

Lay on the ground with your hands placed next to your chest, approximately shoulder-width apart. Push yourself up by straightening your arms and keeping your back straight, or parallel to the ground. This exercise will build and firm your shoulders, arms, and chest.

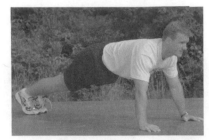

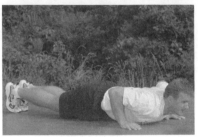

WIDE

From the same position as the regular push-up, place your hands about six to twelve inches away from your chest. You hands should be greater than shoulder-width apart. This slight change in arm distance changes the focus on the muscles being exercised. Now, you are building the chest more than the arms and shoulders.

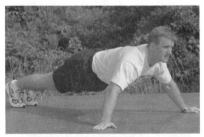

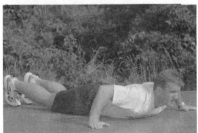

TRICEP

From the same position as the regular push-up, place your hands under your chest about one to two inches away from each other. Spread your legs in order to help with balance. This exercise will concentrate more on the triceps than on the chest.

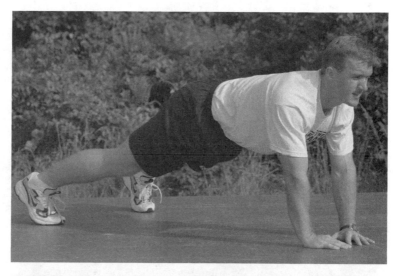

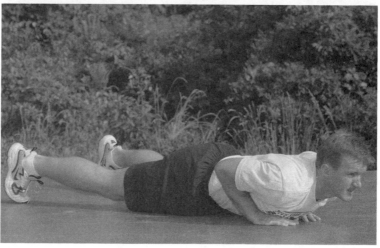

KNEE

If you are having trouble with regular push-ups, or have reached muscle fatigue in your push-up workout, you can always resort to knee push-ups and receive the same muscular benefit. Lay on the ground. With your knees remaining on the ground, lift your body off the floor by straightening your arms and keeping your back stiff.

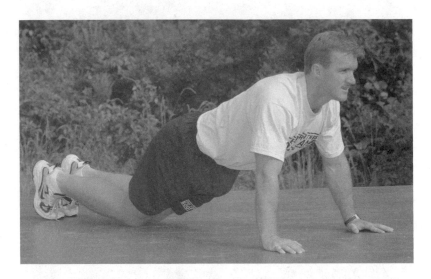

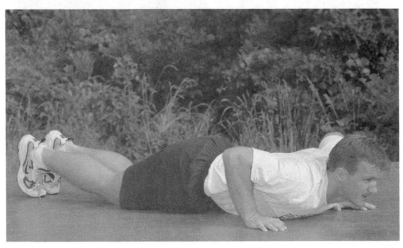

BOX

If knee push-ups are proving to be too difficult, you can lean against a box, chair, or wall and still work the same muscles as regular push-ups.

Facing the object, lean into and catch yourself by placing your arms about shoulder width apart on the object. Bend your arms and touch your chest to the object. Straighten your arms. Before you know it, you will be able to perform knee and regular push-ups.

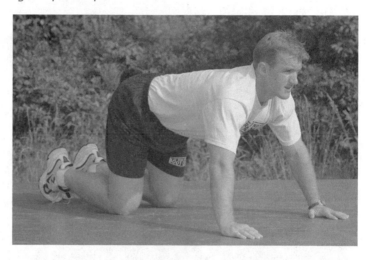

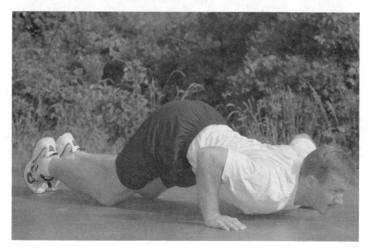

PULL-UPS

REGULAR GRIP

Grab the pull-up bar with your hands placed approximately shoulder width apart and your palms facing away from you. Pull yourself upward until your chin is over the bar and complete the exercise by slowly returning to the hanging position.

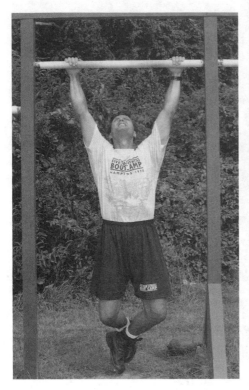 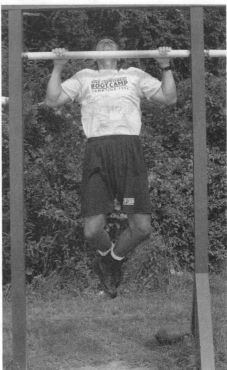

REVERSE GRIP

Grab the pull-up bar with your hands placed approximately two to three inches apart with your palms facing you. Pull yourself upward until your chin is over the bar and complete the exercise by slowly returning to the hanging position.

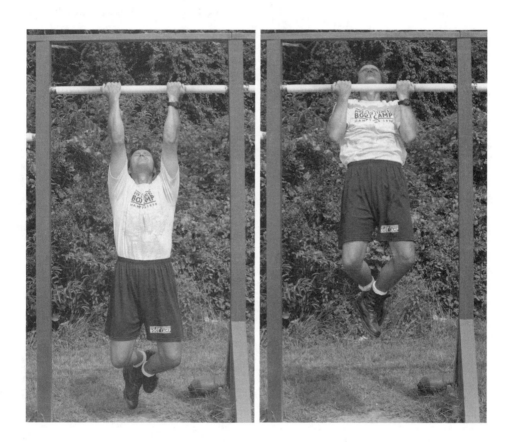

NEGATIVES

If you cannot do any pull-ups, you can do negatives. Negatives are essentially half pull-ups. All you have to do is get your chin over the bar, by standing on a chair for instance.

Then, slowly allow gravity to lower you all the way down, letting your fully-extended arms hang from the bar.

Resist gravity as much as you can—that is what makes this workout tough. Do not put your feet back on the chair and make it easier for yourself. Keep those feet up and fight gravity for a count of five seconds.

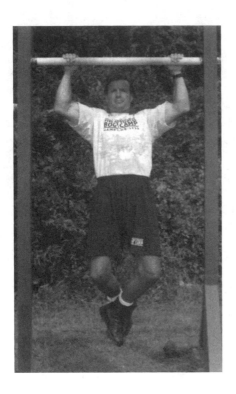 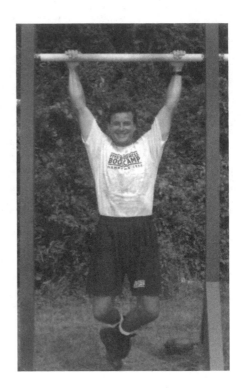

ASSISTED PULL-UPS

A great way to build strength and increase the number of pull-ups you can accomplish, assisted pull-ups are best performed with a workout partner. Grab the pull-up bar with the appropriate grip, cross your ankles, and hang freely. Your workout partner will grab your crossed ankles to provide a stable base, allowing you to use your leg muscles for power through the repetition. Your partner should NOT lift you upward! This can cause leg injuries. Your partner should provide gentle upward pressure below your shoulders to make the pull-up slightly easier while you lift.

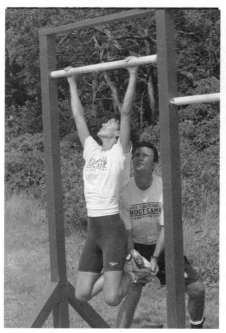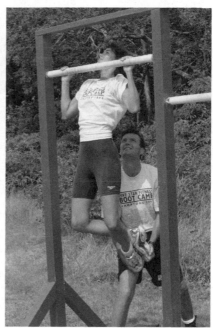

If you are exercising with a partner, you need to communicate the most of your workouts! If you are assisting, do not let go of your partner's ankles without letting them know first! You can seriously injure someone if they are not properly prepared.

STRAIGHT KNEE INCLINES

Using a bar that is three feet off the ground, place yourself under it and grab the bar, using either the regular or reverse grip. Straighten out your back, hips, and legs and pull your chest to the bar. Repeat as required.

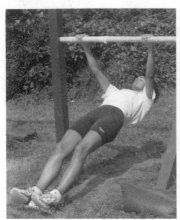 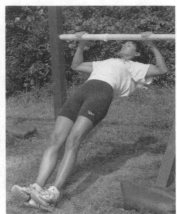

BENT KNEES INCLINES

This is a the mildest possible pull-up. Keep your knees bent and use your leg muscles to lift you through a full range of motion. Gradually, you'll find you can change to the straight inclined pull-up, and before long - full dead hang pull-ups!

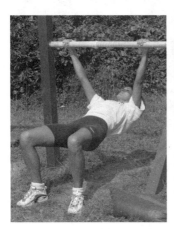 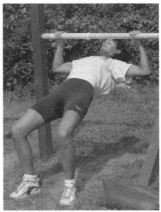

BENCH DIPS

Here is a great tricep (back of arm) exercise. No more wavy underarms if you keep working on this exercise. Simply sit on a chair, bench, or small table. Place your feet about three feet in front of you as you sit on the very edge of the seat. Now, grab the edge of the seat with your hands, lift your butt off the seat, and lower yourself about four to five inches below the seat by bending your arms at the elbow. Straighten your arms and repeat.

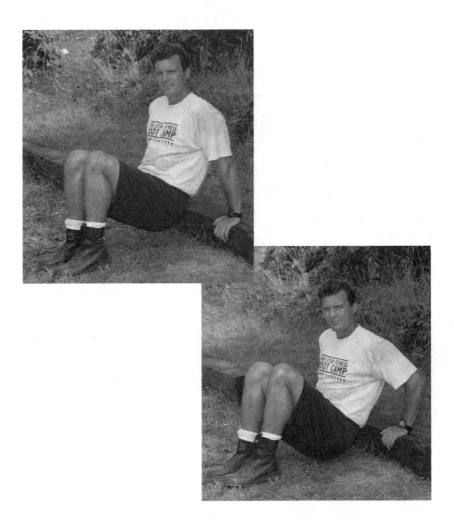

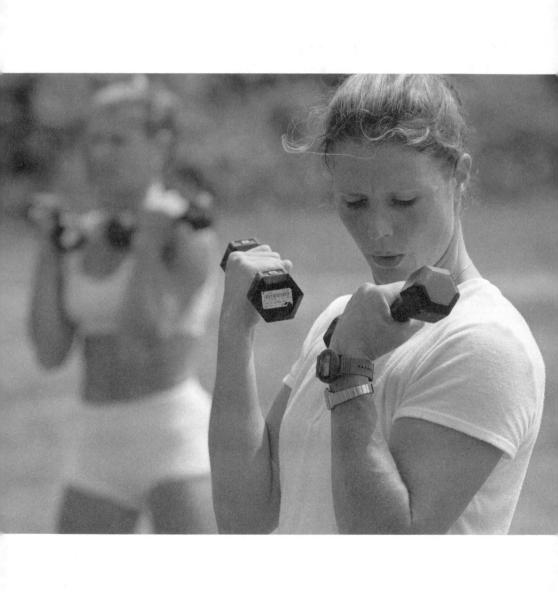

Upper Body
Weight Exercises

For those of you who are afraid of building big, bulging muscles - fear not! The following exercises use resistance training (weights) to build the lean muscle mass required to help burn more calories and fat at rest. You are NOT going to look like a bodybuilder by doing these exercises.

We do not use heavy dumbbells in the weight portion of boot camp because our goal is to build muscle endurance not muscle mass. To accomplish this, you need to do 15 to 25 repetitions with a variety of sets for each muscle group. The objective is to fatigue the muscle group you are exercising. You'll find that after a session of pull-ups, push-ups, and field drills, weights of three to fifteen pounds are more than sufficient. We caution you to observe proper form at all times. Never sacrifice form to lift heavier weights. Be aware of the difference between good and bad pain. Cease any exercise that causes joint pain. Weight training is an essential part of The Five Star Fitness Boot Camp. Whether you're sixteen years old or sixty years old, you'll feel the difference within weeks.

REVERSE FLY

Stand with your feet shoulder width apart, slightly bending your knees. Bend forward at the waist while keeping your back flat. It's important to keep your stomach tight. Let the weights hang by your toes, then lift them outward so they are parallel to your shoulders. Concentrate on squeezing your shoulder blades together. Muscles used: shoulders and upper back.

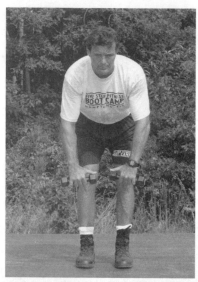

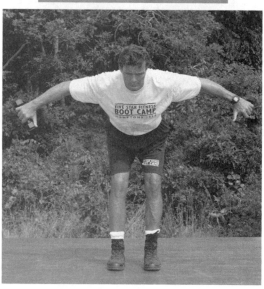

UPRIGHT ROWS

Keep your shoulders back while lifting your elbows chest high. Exhale as you lift. Muscles used: the deltoids (shoulders).

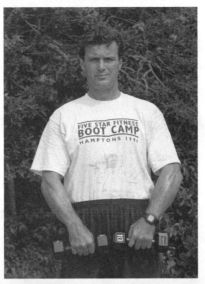

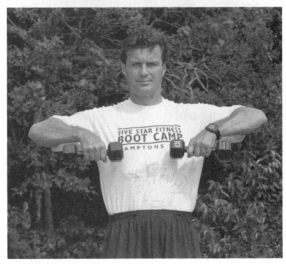

SHOULDER SHRUGS

Hold the weights to your side. Keep your head up and your eyes looking forward. Using a full range of motion, lift your shoulders to your ear. This really helps prevent sloping shoulders and develops and maintains good posture. Muscles used: mid-upper back.

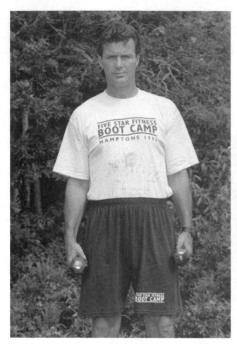

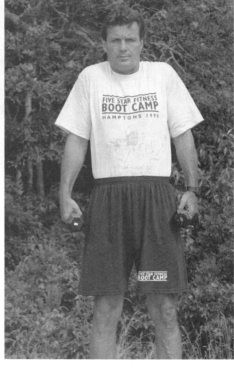

OVERHEAD PRESS (MILITARY PRESS)

An advanced and intensive exercise, start by placing your feet in a staggered stance, with one foot ahead of the other and knees slightly bent to reduce the strain on your lower back. Exhale as you push the weights over your head. Slowly lower them to shoulder height and repeat. Muscles used: shoulders and triceps.

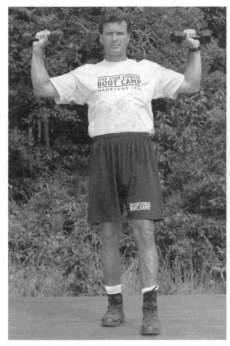

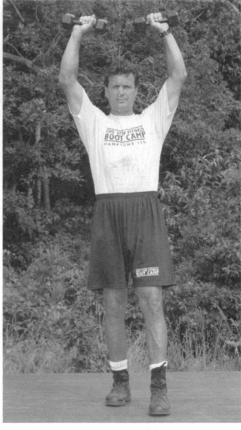

BICEPS CURLS

Hold the weights by your side, fully extending your arms. Slowly bring the weights to your shoulders. Use a complete range of motion and keep this exercise smooth. Do not swing the weights. Nothing should move but your biceps and lungs. Muscles used: biceps.

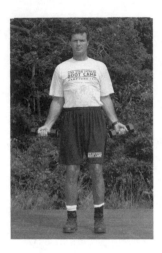 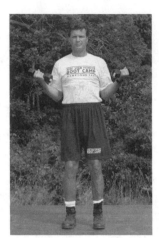

BICEPS "PUMP" (HALF CURLS)

Using lighter weights, work those biceps. These are half repetitions. Leave your arms bent and bring the weights all of the way up to your shoulders, then about half the way down. Then, bring your arms all of the way down, and half the way up. Pump the weights quickly until you feel the burn. Muscles used: biceps.

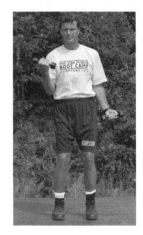 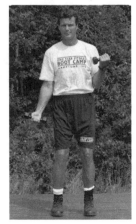

LAWNMOWER – For developing that "V" shaped back, bend forward at waist, let your arms hang fully extended, and pull the weight back to waist height. Keep your trunk stable throughout the full range of motion. Muscles used: back and biceps.

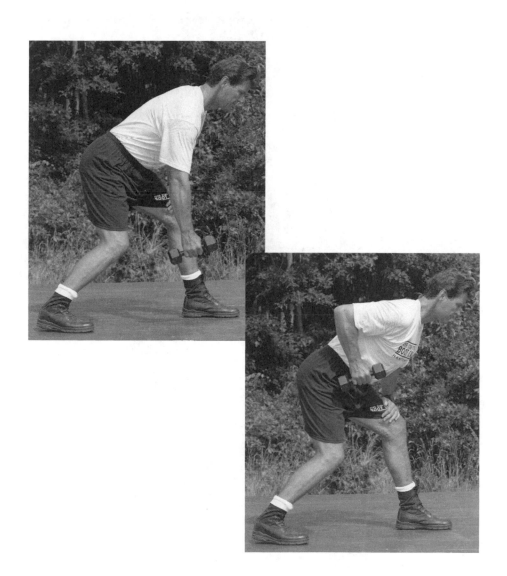

LATERAL RAISE

A safe and effective shoulder exercise, keep your knees slightly bent, shoulder back, and your chest high. Lift weights parallel to ground in a smooth, controlled motion. Muscles used: all shoulder muscles.

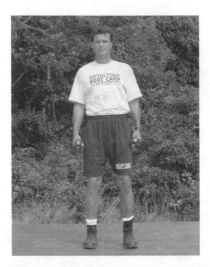

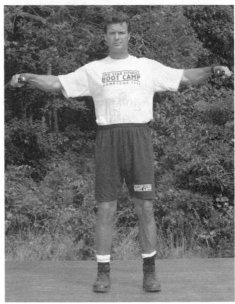

TRICEP EXTENSION

Strong triceps are important to many sports skills. Holding a weight, bring your hands overhead and lower the weight toward the back of your neck. Make certain your elbows remain pointed sky high. Repeat. Muscles used: triceps.

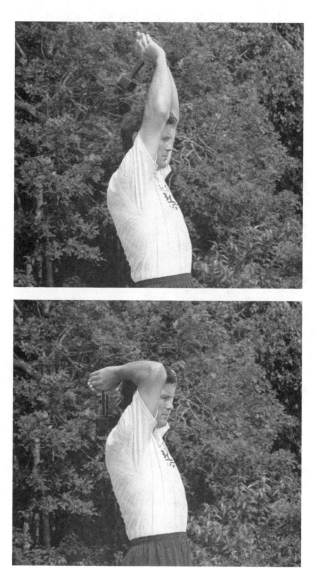

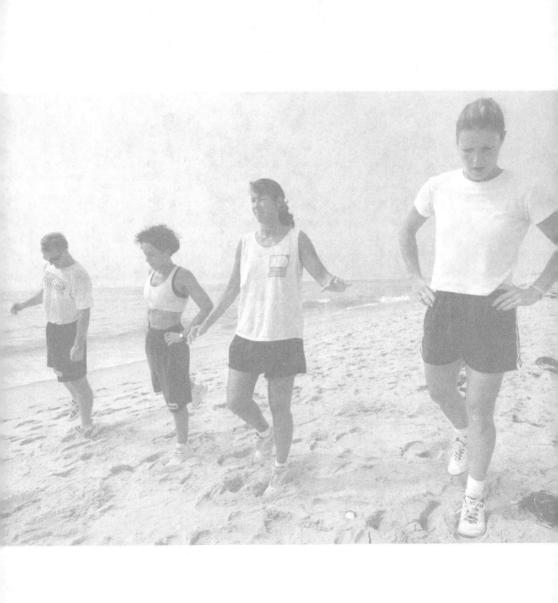

Lower Body
Exercises

The lower body is our foundation of strength. Far more than women, men often fail to grasp this simple fact. What good does it do to have 18 inch biceps and a 44 inch chest if they are being supported by weak and skinny legs? Would you want to live in a house built on swamp land? Our lower body exercises are designed to strengthen the major muscles of the legs, from the butt to the calves.

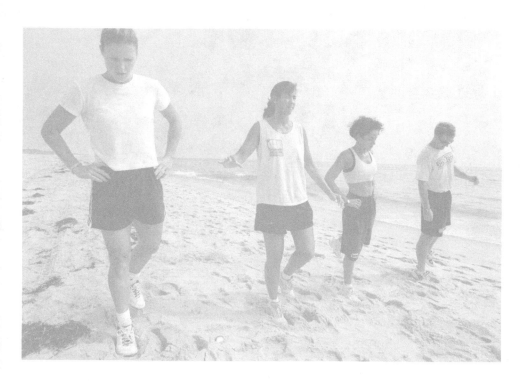

LUNGE

The lunge is a great leg exercise to develop shape and flexibility. It intensifies the work load on the forward leg and requires a greater amount of balance. Keeping your chest up high and your stomach tight, take a long step forward and drop your back knee toward the ground. Stand up on your forward leg, bringing your feet together and repeat with the other leg. Muscles used: upper and lower legs, and butt.

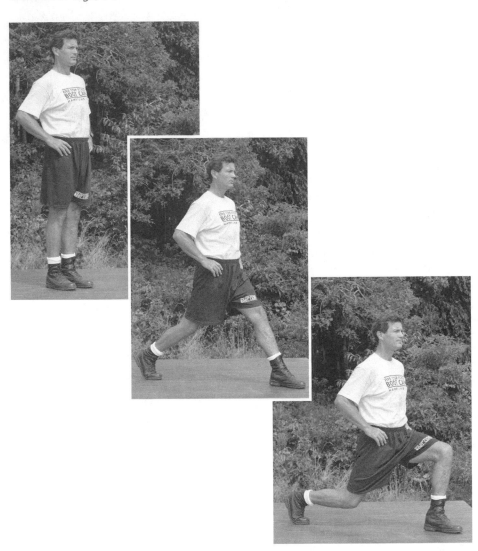

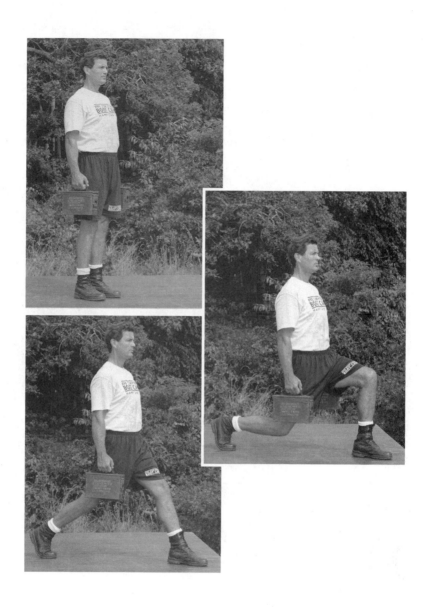

Want to make your lunges more challenging? Grab some weights, or ammo cans filled with sand, and perform numerous repetitions.

LUNGES (ON LOGS OR STEPS)

A spicy version of the regular lunge, this frontal leg assault develops defined and strong quadriceps. Maintain good posture while allowing the forward leg to do most of the work. Remember to keep your forward foot directly under your knee and to breathe. Muscles used: quadriceps, hamstrings, and glutes (legs and butt).

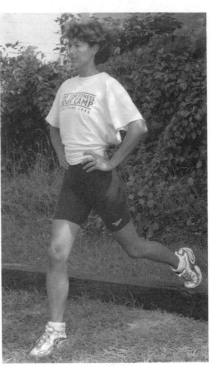

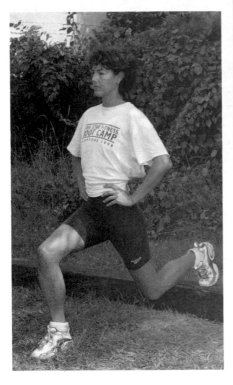

HIGH KNEE KICK ON LOG

Time to join the Rockettes! This exercise is fabulous for the quads and abs. Start with one leg on the log and the other behind you on the ground. Kick your back leg forward, bringing your knee up as you squeeze your abs. Rise up on the stationary leg, keeping your balance with your arms. Feel the force in your stomach and forward leg. Repeat and reverse leg positions to target the opposite quadricep. Muscles used: calves, quadriceps, and abdominals.

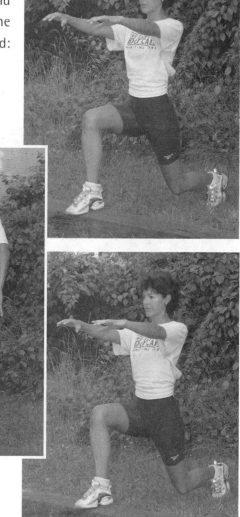

SQUATS

Keeping your feet shoulder width apart, drop your butt back as though sitting in a chair. Concentrate on squeezing your glutes in an upward motion. Keep your heels solid on the ground. Muscles used: glutes, quadriceps, and hamstrings.

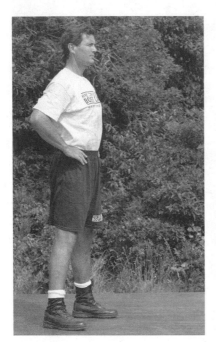

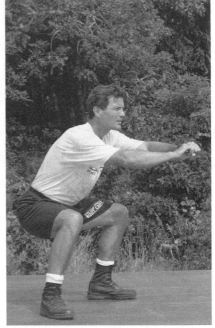

Intensify your squat by posting. While in the full squat position, hold the pose and alternate up and down within a six inch range of motion, similar to riding a horse.

CALF RAISE

This exercise belongs in everyone's arsenal. Hook one foot behind the other and raise up on your toes. Make certain you use a full range of motion. It won't take long to make this burn. Muscles used: calves.

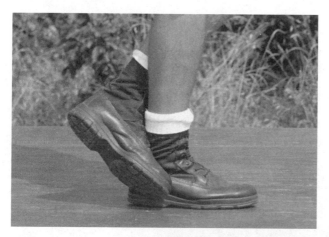

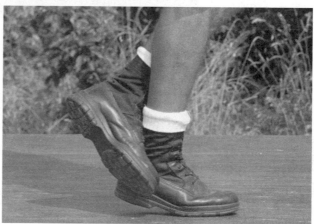

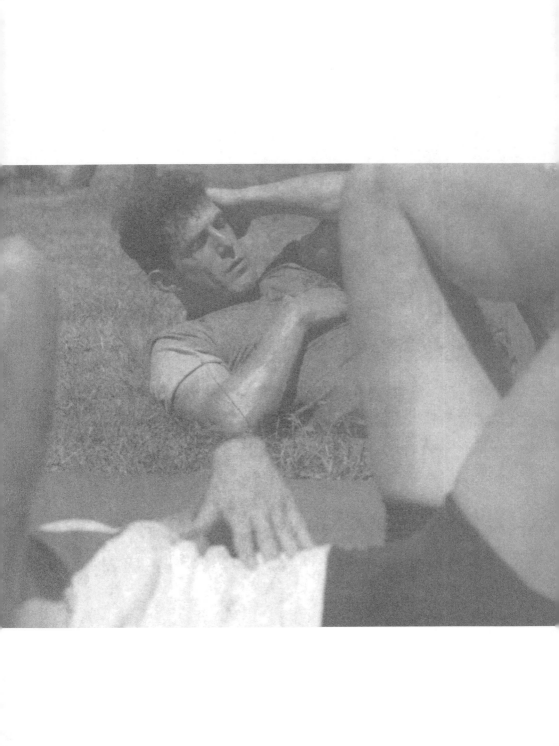

Abdominal Exercises

The major abdominal exercise used in the Boot Camp Workout is the crunch. You will perform crunches eight different ways: regular, reverse, left, right, and the advanced of these four. Adding a few more abdominal exercises and a couple of lower back stretches will firm up a soft belly.

REMEMBER: When you exercise your stomach muscles, be sure to exercise and stretch your back as well. The stomach and lower back muscles are opposing muscle groups and if one is much stronger than the other, you can easily injure the weaker muscle group.

REGULAR CRUNCH

Lay on your back with your feet and knees bent in the air. Cross your hands over your chest and bring your elbows to your knees by flexing your stomach.

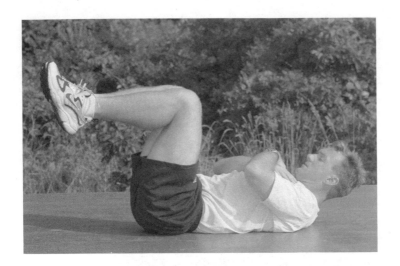

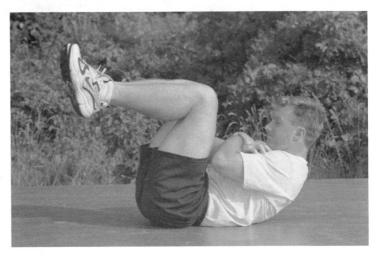

REVERSE CRUNCH

In the same position as the regular crunch, lift your knees and butt toward your elbows, leaving your head and upper body flat on the ground. Only move your legs and butt.

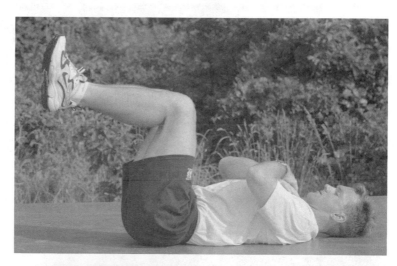

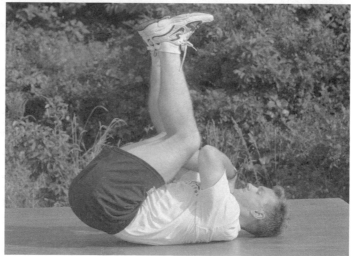

RIGHT ELBOW TO LEFT KNEE

Cross your left leg over your right leg. Flex your stomach and twist to bring your right elbow to your left knee.

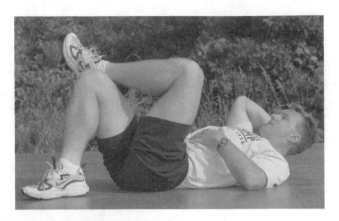

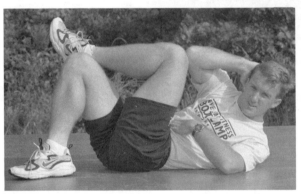

LEFT ELBOW TO RIGHT KNEE

Cross your right leg over your left leg. Flex your stomach and twist to bring your left elbow to your right knee.

ADVANCED CRUNCH (LEGS UP)

Laying on your back, keep your feet straight up in the air. Cross your hands over your chest and bring your elbows to your knees by flexing your stomach.

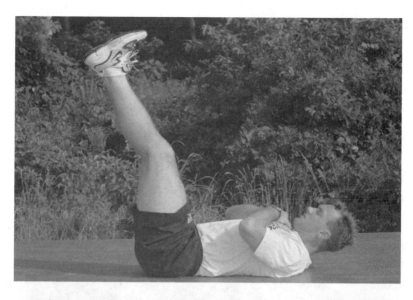

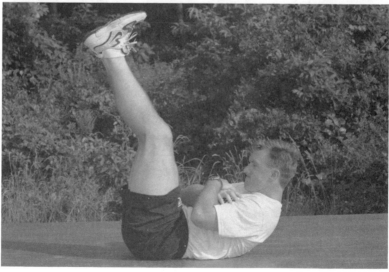

ADVANCED REVERSE (LEGS UP)

Leaving your upper body flat on the ground, lay on your back and lift your butt and legs straight into the air by flexing the lower abdominal region.

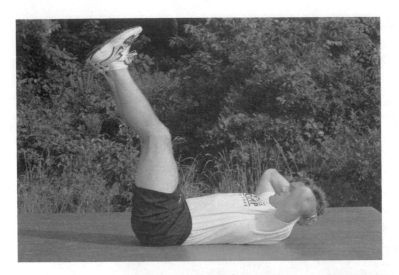

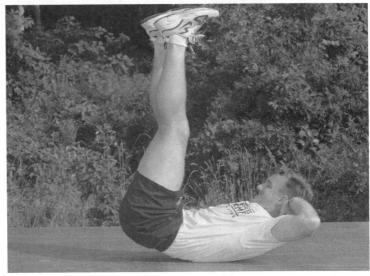

ADVANCED RIGHT ELBOW TO LEFT KNEE (LEG UP)

Crossing your left leg over your right leg, lift your right leg straight into the air. Bring your right elbow to your left knee by flexing your stomach and twisting to the left.

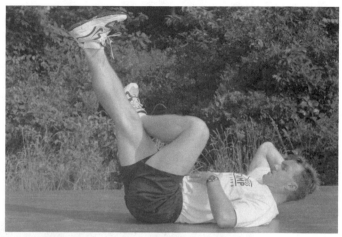

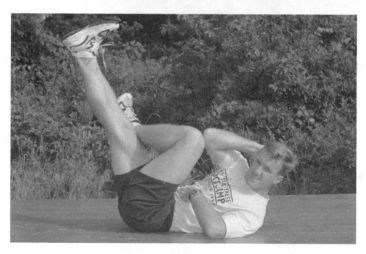

ADVANCED LEFT ELBOW TO RIGHT KNEE (LEG UP)

Crossing your right leg over your left leg, lift your left leg straight into the air. Bring your left elbow to your right knee by flexing your stomach and twisting to the right.

BUTT WIGGLE

Lay on your back with your feet and knees in the air and your knees bent. Keeping your upper body still, wiggle your hips to the left and right and shake your butt.

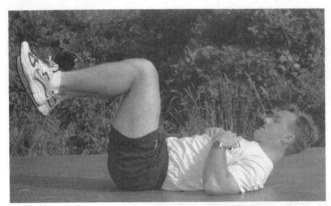

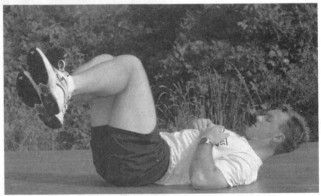

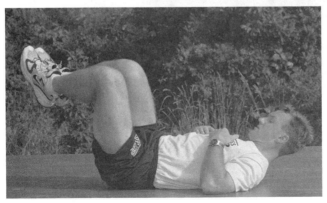

SIDE OBLIQUE

Laying on your right side, lift your legs about three inches off the ground and hold them there. Lift your shoulder about three inches off the ground and repeat. Switch sides and work the other love handle.

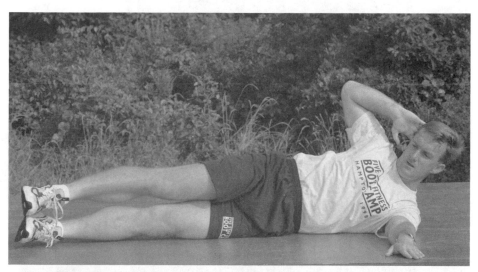

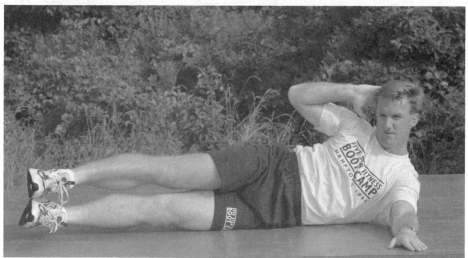

PRONE LOWER BACK EXERCISE

Lay on your stomach with your arms extended over your head. Lift your right arm and your left leg off the ground at the same time. Switch arms/legs and repeat.

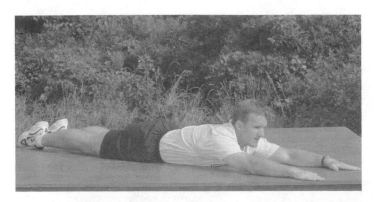

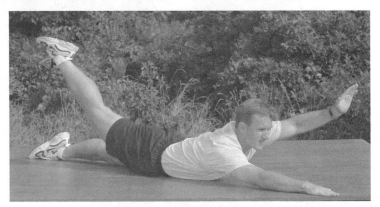

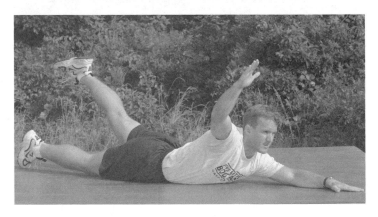

LOWER BACK EXERCISE # 2

On your hands and knees, lift your right arm and your left leg off the ground and extend them. Switch arms/legs and repeat.

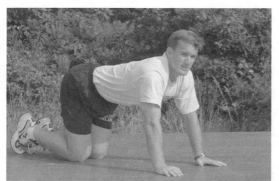

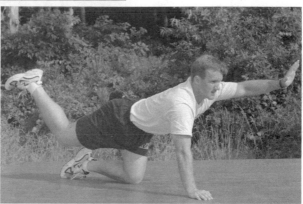

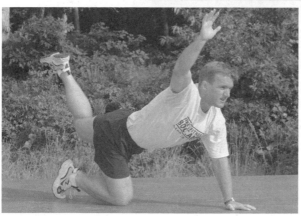

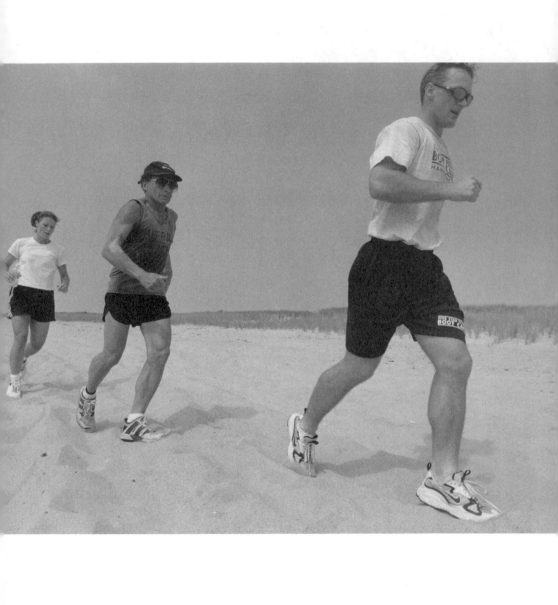

Beach Drills

Beach Drills

On alternate days of the Boot Camp Workout, we concentrated on lower body and cardiovascular exercises. A great workout for the legs and lungs is a run on the beach. The soft sand adds a little more difficulty when running. We recommend stepping into previously made depressions in the sand—footprints, tire tracks, etc. You will definitely feel the thighs, hamstrings, and calf muscles working extra hard while running on this soft surface.

After a mile and a half of running, stop for a water break. After a few minutes, pick things back up with lower body calisthenic exercises such as squats, lunges, calf raises, and frog hops (broad jumps). After burning out your legs with calisthenics, you have to run back to our starting point—another mile and a half!

CALF RAISES

Calf raises (heel raises, actually) are great exercises for developing the lower part of the leg and strengthening the ankles. To do this exercise on the beach, you need to find firm footing and rise up onto the balls of your feet for 20 to 25 repetitions. Alternate each leg, performing the single leg version of this exercise for more difficulty. If you are a beginner, perform this with both feet firmly on the ground, making it a little easier on your ankles and calf muscles.

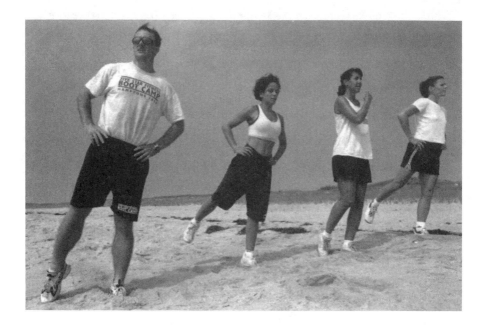

LUNGE

Take a big step with either foot. Bend both knees, keeping your front knee directly over your ankle during the deepest part of the bend. DO NOT EXTEND THE KNEE OVER THE ANKLE—this will cause severe stress on your knee joint and can result in possible injury. Keep your front shin perpendicular to the ground as much as possible. Do these exercises slowly and deliberately. Keep repeating your steps until you have completed 10 to 15 lunges on each leg.

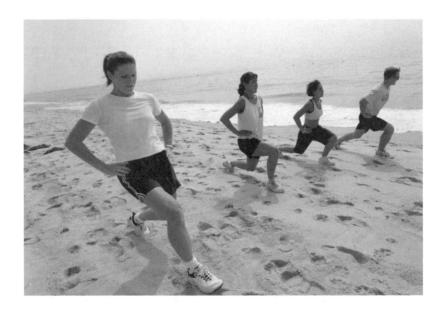

FROG HOPS (BROAD JUMPS)

This exercise is definitely an advanced workout and is not recommended for beginners. Always do your jumps on a soft surface like the beach, grass, or foam rubber mats. DO NOT JUMP ON HARD SURFACES LIKE ASPHALT OR CONCRETE. The impact of landing can cause injury IF done improperly or on improper surfaces.

To complete a "frog hop," simply squat and jump forward as far as you can. Repeat for a total of 5 to 10 jumps. This will build explosive power in your legs and aid in reducing your sprint times and increasing your vertical leap.

Always remember to stretch before, during, and after a leg workout program like this one. Your lower back and legs may be more sore than normal after running on such a soft surface. Once again, stretch and do a few sets of lower back exercises to help ease the soreness.

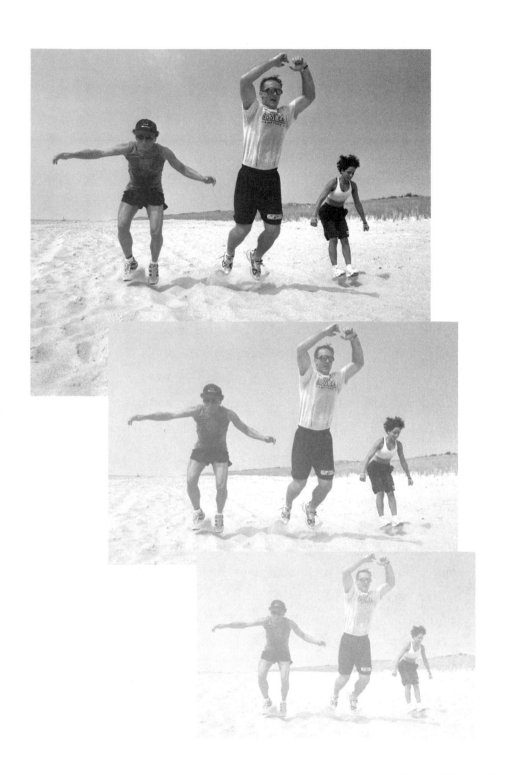

Field Drills and Sprints

Speed play is the name of the game here. Field Drills enhance power, agility, balance, speed, and coordination while increasing aerobic endurance. These drills can be adapted to a wide range of fitness levels, from beginners to highly trained athletes. Give your body time to adjust to these exercises and remember, no one in the history of the world has ever achieved total fitness in one single workout!

A type of training developed in eastern Europe and discovered and refined in the United States in the early 70's and 80's, plyometric exercises are used by both serious athletes and weekend warriors. Plyometrics give people increased body control and balance. They are high impact exercises and should be used with diligence and planning.

To understand plyometrics, you need to know something about how muscles work. Muscles have both lengthening contractions (eccentric motion) and shortening contractions (concentric motion). These contractions work together and individually to help you move. Muscles react to your changes of speed and direction. The quicker they react, the more balance and agility we develop. Plyometrics conditions this reaction time to make it as quick as possible.

For the Boot Camp Workout, we use a variety of plyometric drills for both the Upper and Lower Body. Begin at a low impact level, making sure you land lightly on your toes. The plyometic portion of your workout should always be at the start or during the middle of your exercise routine. Allow plenty of time to recover between sets because fatigue often causes injury.

Plyometrics add variety and spice to workouts and can easily be part of a circuit training workout which includes sprinting, hopping, and skipping. Keep intensity and duration low. As conditioning increases, add volume and intensity.

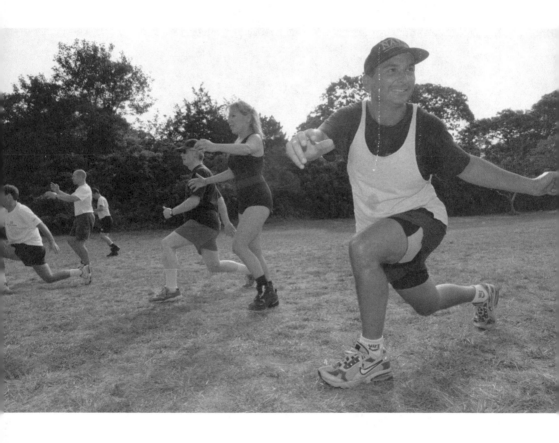

THE GOOSE STEP

Keeping your legs straight, kick as high as your waist while reaching your opposite hand toward your toe. Keep your stomach tight throughout this drill.

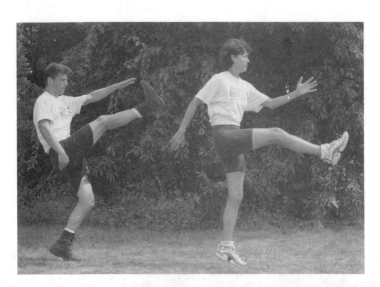

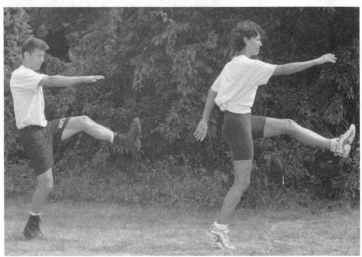

SKIPPING

Just like when you were in kindergarten, skipping is a great warm-up or cool down exercise. Plus, it's guaranteed to put a smile on your face.

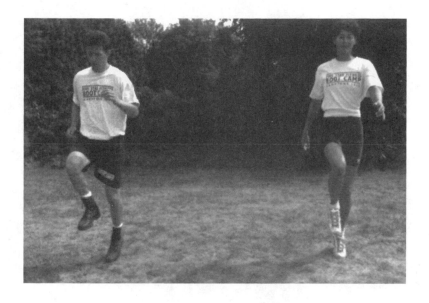

POWER SKIP OR HOP

This move will really get your heart pumping! Bring your knees up to your chest. This drill can be done while moving forward or standing in place. Start slowly then work toward building speed as you maintain high knee action.

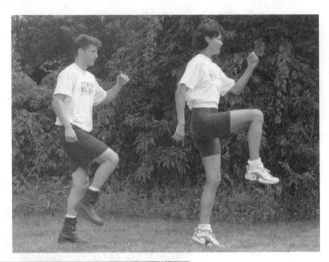

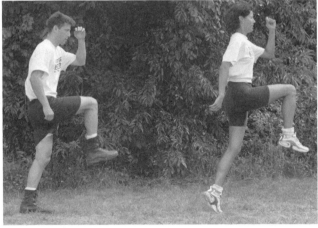

THE KARIOKE

Start by standing shoulder width apart. While moving left, step your right leg in front of your left leg. Bring your legs apart. On the next move, bring your right leg behind your left leg. Keep moving to the left throughout this drill for the specified distance. When moving to the right, reverse the sequence by crossing your left leg in front of and then behind your right leg. Start these slowly, then pick up the pace.

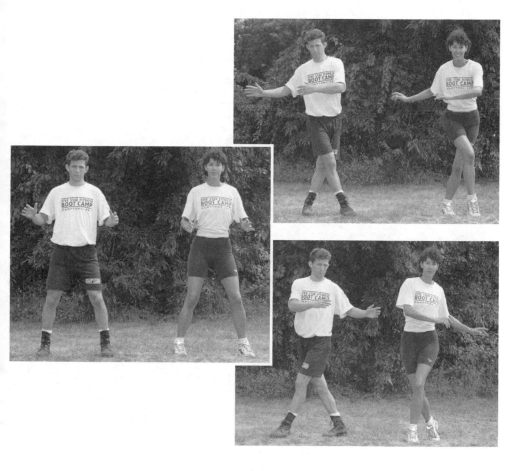

PIZZA LUNGE

Requiring concentration and coordination, this drill works the legs, butt, and abs all in one (and works off those pizza pie lunches).

This exercise is performed as a regular moving lunge, with a twist. As you lunge forward and down, twist your trunk to the side of your forward knee while swinging your arms as if you were carrying a pizza. Then lunge forward on the other leg, twisting your body to the other side.

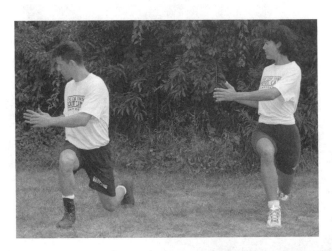

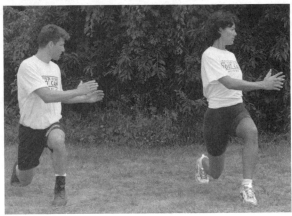

HIGH KNEE KICK

Another great plyometric field exercise, lift your knees high in rapid succession—left-right-left-right—while swinging your arms. These can be done in place or slowly moving forward. Just keep focused on lifting your knees as high as possible!

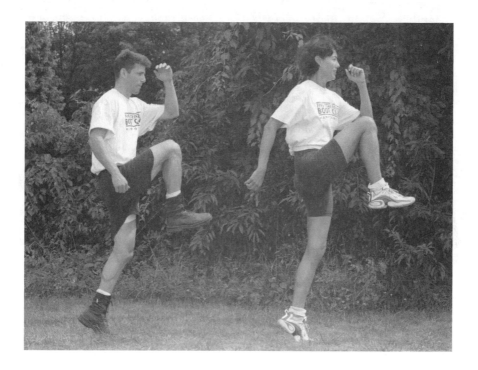

SPRINTING TECHNIQUES TO BECOME FASTER

To become a faster short distance runner use the following techniques in your Field Drills training:

1) **Explosive starts**—When you begin running, stay low for the first 5 to 10 yards and lean forward, taking short steps as you accelerate. Standing straight up at the start of your sprint will slow you down immediately.

2) **Lean forward and pump those arms**—In short distances, such as 20 to 100 yard sprints, leaning forward and pumping your arms quickly will help increase your speed.

3) **Shift into second gear**—After 10 yards, it is time to change gears. This is when you will pop up, stick your chest out, pump those arms hard, and lengthen your stride.

4) **Breathing**—When you are running as fast as you can, you naturally have to breathe. Your breaths should be quick inhales and quick exhales, unlike the big, deep breaths you take when you are jogging.

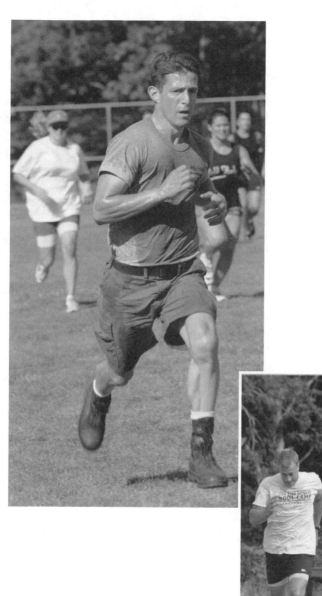

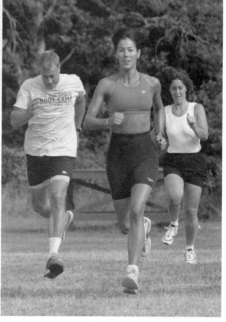

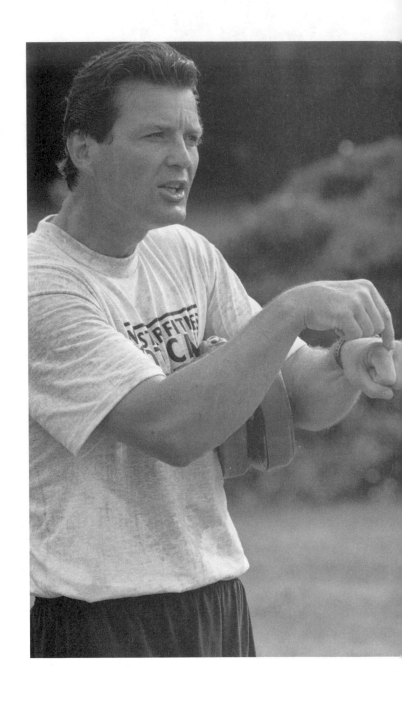

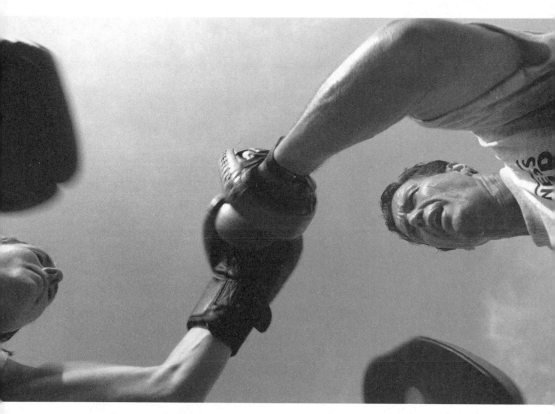

Cross Training
with
Basic Boxing

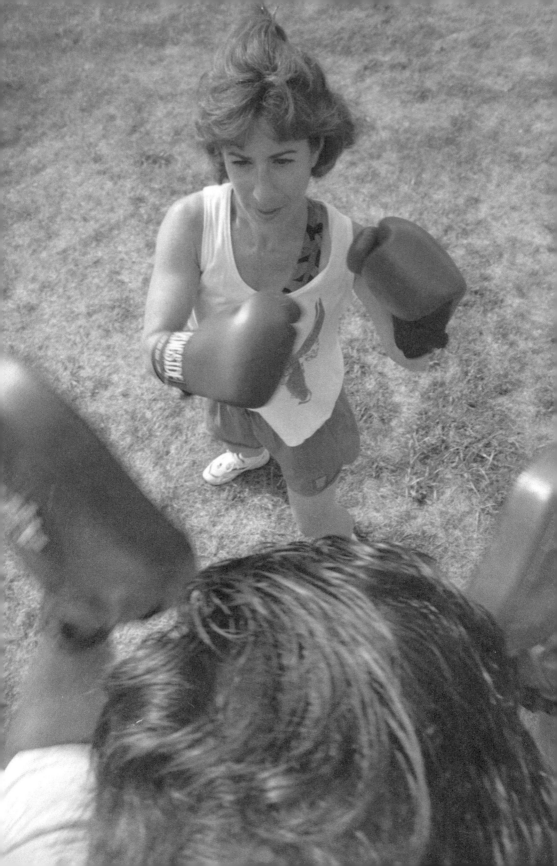

Boxing Basics

Boxing Basics

Boxing drills are a sure-fire way to improve your cardiovascular system, increase lean body mass, and burn tons of calories. Always crowd-pleasers at Boot Camp, especially with a Golden Gloves Champ in the ring, we added them to the workout on days when participants just did not feel like running. Boxing drills are fantastic cross-training tools for those of you eager to be challenged. Try them once a week or so to add an exciting dimension to your workout regimen.

A few basic instructions must be followed for safe training:

- For properly protection, you must first wrap and glove your hands and wrists.

- Keep your wrists straight and make certain that contact is made only on your second and third knuckles.

- By shadow boxing, you do not need to tape your hands and you still get a great workout.

Shadow Boxing

The most underrated exercise in boxing, shadow boxing is simply boxing against an imaginary opponent. This is a terrific way to practice your offensive and defensive movements. Concentration is the key in this exercise. Begin slowly and increase speed as your skills improve.

LEFT JAB

If there is one punch you ought to learn, it should be the jab. Jabbing gives you timing, distance, and is the foundation for punching in combinations.

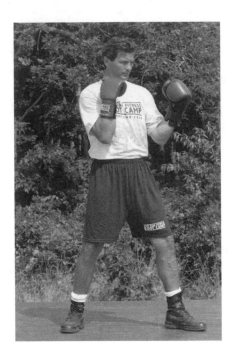

1. Assume the "on guard' position by keeping your feet shoulder width apart, knees bent, elbows to your waist, and hands by your cheeks. Take a step forward with your left foot and point your right foot towards three o'clock. Balance is key. Let your energy rock you gently from foot to foot.

Remember: throwing a punch is basically shifting your body weight from one foot to the other.

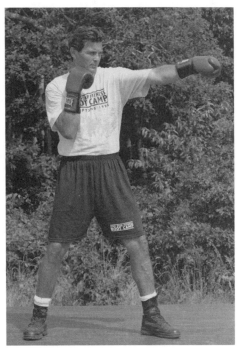

2. As your weight shifts from your right foot to your left, extend your left arm out and back as quickly as possible. BAM! BAM! BAM! Be careful not to hyperextend or "snap" your elbow joint. Begin slowly and as you develop "muscle memory," pick up the pace.

Muscle memory is way of describing the fact that your body will grow increasingly comfortable with new exercises over time.

THE RIGHT CROSS

Bring on the heat! The right cross is a punch thrown with your power hand— your right hand if you're right-handed, your left if you're left-handed. To throw a good straight right cross, there are three things you must do.

1. Make sure you pivot your right foot when throwing the punch.

2. Keep your knees bent.

3. Put your weight behind it.

   KAPOW!

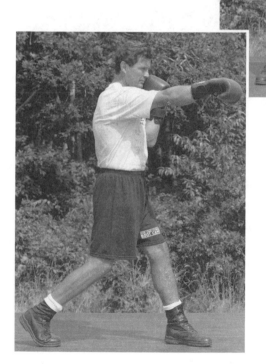

THE LEFT HOOK

The left hook is the toughest punch to throw in boxing, yet when executed properly, it is the most effective.

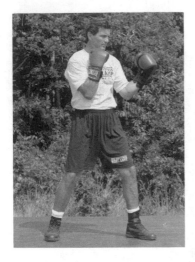

1. Start in the "on guard" position.

2. Anchor your right foot, pressing down and pivoting on the ball of your left foot (see the picture below). At the same time, turn your left hip, lift your left elbow to shoulder height with your palm facing you, and . . . BAM! Left hook!

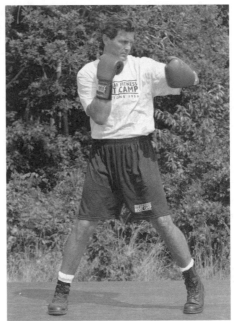

THE BOB

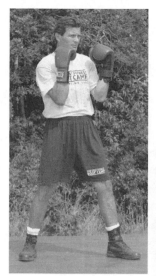

1. Start in the "on guard" position.

2. Sit straight down as if you were sitting in a chair.

3. Stand straight up to resume the starting "on guard" position.

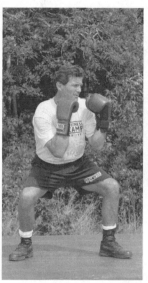 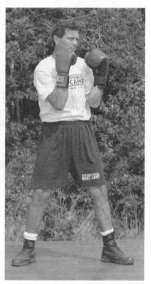

The Weave

1. From the sitting position of the bob, shift your body weight over your right foot so that your head is positioned over your right knee and stand up!

2. To bob and weave to the right, repeat the movement over the left knee.

3. If you bob and weave to the left, your weight is on the your left side allowing you to implement a left hook. When you bob and weave over the right, you can use a right cross. Whichever side your weight is on is your power side.

THE DUCK WALK

For a more advanced workout, this drill will help you learn to use the leg muscles needed to generate power. This is a moving drill.

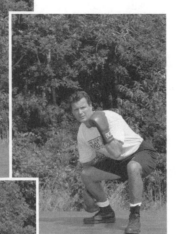

1. Start in the "on guard" position.

2. Sit down and touch your right shoe with your right glove, keeping your left glove at your cheek.

3. Stand up, pivot your right foot and turn at the hip while extending your right hand and . . . POW! Right Cross!

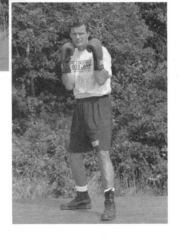

4. Return to the "on guard" position.

5. Step forward with your right foot.

6. Repeat the same motions with your left hand.

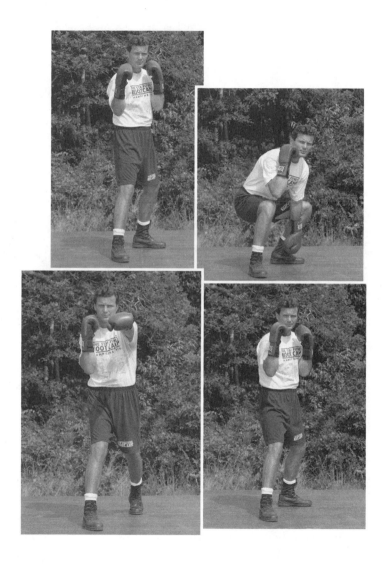

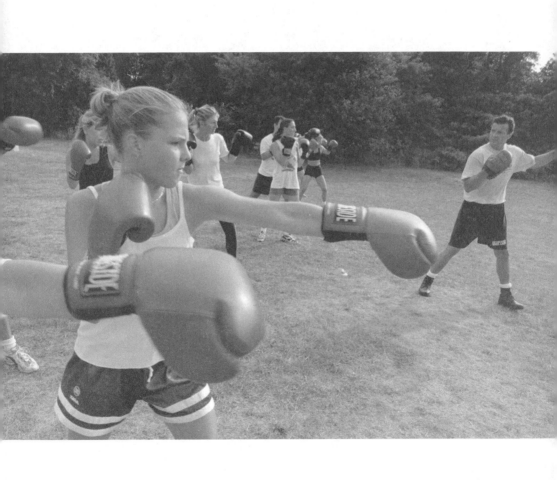

Main Event

Main Event Workout

Six weeks to main event

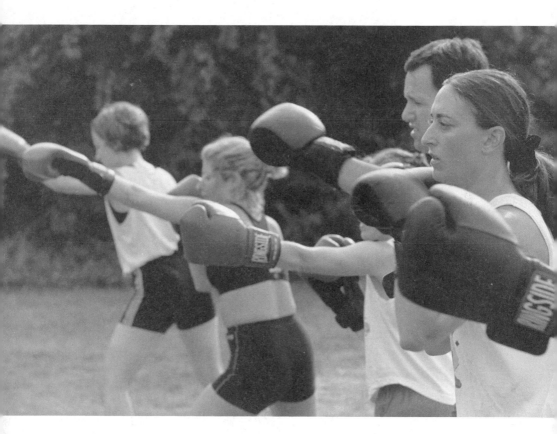

GOLDEN GLOVES—*Weeks one and two*

These exercises are ten rounds, three minutes each in length, with one minute rests between rounds. Start with one push-up, adding one push-up per round during the rest periods. Use slow, controlled movements to develop muscle memory and skill. Be careful to avoid snapping your elbows or shoulders.

Round 1:   skip rope
           1 push-up

Round 2:   stretch
           2 push-ups

Round 3:   shadow box—jab
           3 push-ups

Round 4:   shadow box—jab/cross
           4 push-ups

Round 5:   shadow box—jab/cross/hook
           5 push-ups

Round 6:   shadow box—jab/cross/hook/cross/jab
           6 push-ups

Round 7:   shadow box—bob and weave
           7 push-ups

Round 8:   lower back exercises
           8 push-ups

Round 9:   main event three-minute abs (see inset on page 99)
           9 push-ups

Round 10: stretch

PROFESSIONAL—*Weeks three and four*

By the third week, your speed of movement should increase. Be careful not to sacrifice technique. Start with five push-ups between rounds.

Round 1:   skip rope
5 push-ups

Round 2:   stretch
6 push-ups

Round 3:   skip rope, interval speed (15 seconds high, 15 seconds low)
7 push-ups

Round 4:   shadow box—jab/cross
8 push-ups

Round 5:   shadow box—jab/cross/hook
9 push-ups

Round 6:   shadow box—jab/cross/hook/bob and weave
10 push-ups

Round 7:   shadow box—jab/cross/hook/cross/hook
11 push-ups

Round 8:   five single leg lunges on each leg
12 push-ups

Round 9:   main event abs
13 push-ups

Round 10:   lower back exercises
10 minutes of stretching

THE MAIN EVENT—*Weeks four and five*

You are now prime time. Pick up the speed and add power.

Round 1: skip rope
10 push-ups

Round 2: skip rope intervals (30 seconds high, 30 seconds low)
11 push-ups

Round 3: shadow box—double jab/cross
double jab/cross/hook
double jab/cross/hook/cross
12 push-ups

Round 4: shadow box—double jab/cross
double jab/cross/jab/cross/hook
13 push-ups

Round 5: shadow box—double jab/cross/hook/bob and weave
14 push-ups

Round 6: shadow box—double jab/hook/cross
double jab/bob and weave/cross
double jab/bob and weave/hook
15 push-ups

Round 7: shadow box—double jab/bob and weave/hook/cross/hook
double jab/bob and weave/cross/hook/cross
16 push-ups

Round 8: 10 squats/jumping jacks for 30 seconds
17 push-ups

Round 9:   lower back exercises for 30 seconds
           back extenders for 30 seconds
           18 push-ups

Round 10: main event abs
           cool down 10 minute stretch

Main Event Abs—The Three Minute Gut Buster!

—25 crunches
—25 reverse crunches
—25 right crunches
—25 right obliques
—25 left crunches
—25 left obliques
—25 reverse crunches

—25 opposite elbow-opposite knee
—50 bicycles-controlled motion extending legs out, opposite elbow-opposite knee
—50 butt wiggles

If you have back problems, keep your feet on the ground during the ab routine.

These exercises flow smoothly from one to the other. Make sure your abs stay tight during the whole cycle.

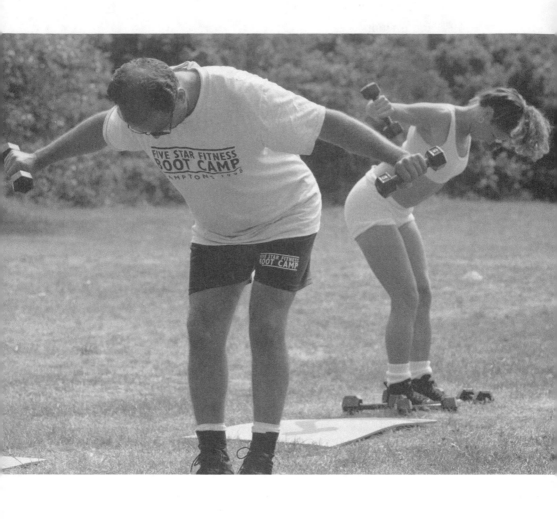

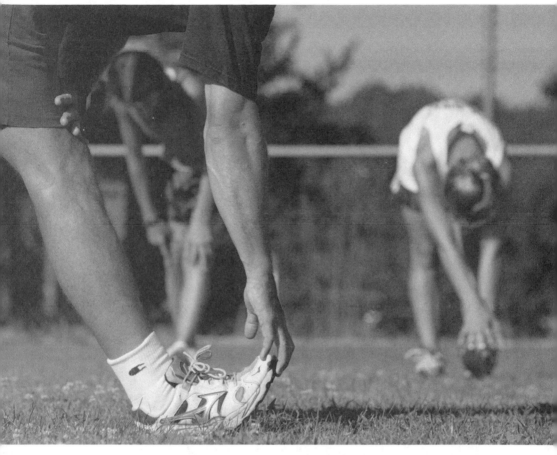

Part III

The Official Boot Camp Workout Schedules

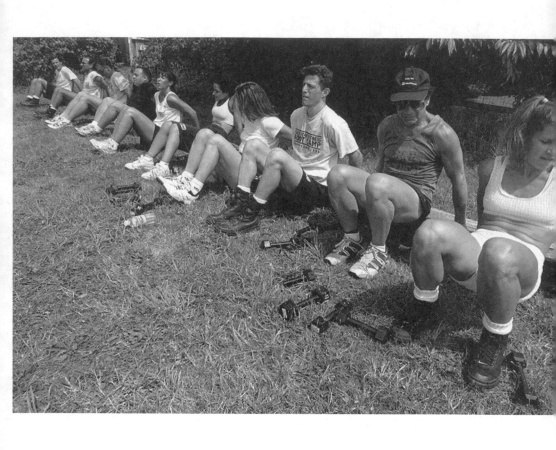

Workouts

Workouts

In the Official Five Star Fitness Boot Camp Workout, there are over 20 different workouts with over 50 different exercises. Understandably, these workouts could confuse the most avid exerciser, let alone a beginner. So, this chapter is dedicated to explaining our workouts, just as the previous chapters explained individual exercises and stretches.

*Remember to stretch well before and after these workouts. Muscle pulls or tears are common if one is not properly stretched.

Sets x Reps Concept:

Throughout the following pages of workouts, you will see the phrase "sets x reps." This is a common term in the fitness world that abbreviates the word, repetitions.

It simply means you will repeat a certain number of exercises a certain number of times. For example, when instructed to do 3 x 10 Banch Dips, you would do 10 repetitions of dips a total of three times.

Whenever you see "set x reps" in these workouts, give yourself 30 to 60 seconds rest before you start up the next set.

THE PULL-UP WORKOUT

Pull-ups are the greatest upper body exercise around! For the pull-up workout, grab the pull-up bar and pull yourself over the bar as shown in the exercise chapter (page 32). Simply start off the workout with one pull-up. Get off the bar and stretch for about 30 seconds and do the next set—two pull-ups. You will want to rest between pull-up sets for no longer than one minute. Continue the pull-ups until you cannot perform any more—THEN resort to negatives for the remainder of the workout.

A word about negatives for those who cannot do pull-ups: Many men and women cannot perform any pull-ups. The only reason you cannot do a pull-up is probably because you do not practice doing pull-ups. So, for the majority of you who have not done pull-ups in years or have never done pull-ups, this workout will challenge you. Step up to the bar and take that challenge!

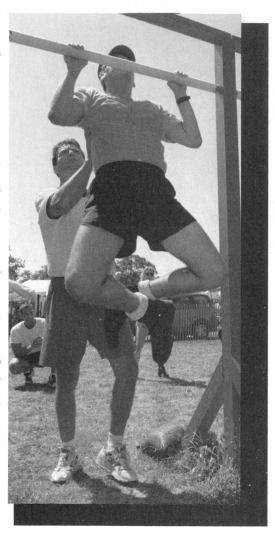

Do the specified number of repetitions as directed by the Five Star Fitness Bootcamp Workout and soon you will be able to pull yourself over that bar.

Perform the same repetitions with the reverse grip pull-ups after you have finished the regular grip pull-up.

PUSH-UP / CRUNCH SUPERSET

This is a great way to achieve extraordinary repetitions of push-ups and crunches! Each of the six sets of exercises should be completed within a two minute period. For example:

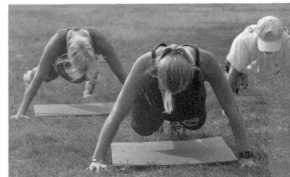

Set #1—Two minutes!
8 regular push-ups
8 regular crunches
8 wide push-ups
8 reverse crunches
8 triceps push-ups
8 ½ sit-ups

You should finish early sets with at least 30 to 45 seconds remaining. Use this time to stretch or drink some water. You will repeat this particular workout eight times. Total time should only be 16 minutes, BUT you will achieve almost 200 push-ups and 200 abdominal exercises in that time! Sound impossible? I promise you it is not!

Rest: There is no rest time while on the two minute clock. Do your set as quickly as possible, but watch your form. Do not jeopardize your form for a faster superset time. This is a great time saver workout if you are too busy to take 30 to 45 minutes to exercise. Take 10 to 20 minutes and be amazed at yourself performing 100 to 200 push-ups and crunches in that time.

AB / LOWER BACK EXERCISES

During the beginning few weeks of this workout cycle, you will only do one set of the following abdominal / lower back exercises:

Four-way crunches
Half sit-ups
Butt wiggles
Back exercises #1 and #2.

Do *not* rest in between exercises. However, you can do an abdominal stretch for 15 seconds if you need to.

During the advanced workouts (medium/spicy), you will run through the exercises twice. A four-way crunch is usually the most confusing exercise of this workout. Quite simply, it is an abbreviation for doing four different types of crunches—regular, reverse, left, and right.

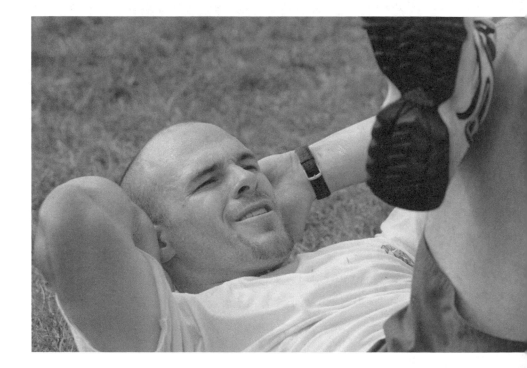

DUMBBELL PT WORKOUT

You have seen the descriptions of the weight exercises. Now, this is how you put it all together. You will only perform the exercises for one set of 8 reps. There is no rest between exercises. Go through this workout nonstop giving yourself an enormous upper body pump. At the end of the last exercise in the sequence (lawnmowers), you can drop the weights and rest before you perform the 2 sets x 8 reps of biceps curls.

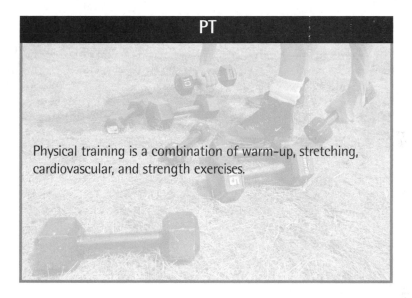

PT

Physical training is a combination of warm-up, stretching, cardiovascular, and strength exercises.

LOWER BODY PT

There will be three exercises you will perform on lower body PT days: squats, lunges, and calf raises.

This workout can be accomplished one of two ways:

1) Alternating sets—Perform the required reps of squats, then lunges, then calf raises. After completing the first set of each exercise, take a minute to rest before beginning the second. Repeat if required.

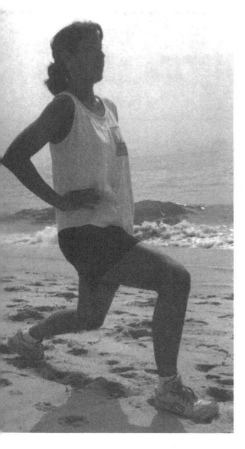

2) Regular sets—Perform the required number of squat repititions. Take a 30 second rest, then repeat the squats again until all sets are completed. Move onto lunges the same way, then finish with calf raises.

*You can use dumbbells to increase the difficulty of this workout.

FIELD DRILLS

These workouts are probably the hardest workouts to do on your own with intensity. If you follow the program and rest for the allotted time and no more, you will receive a cardiovascular workout like no other. Though it is difficult to keep up the intensity on your own, it is quite easy to follow. Simply begin the field drills with the first exercise and follow in the flow chart below.

The workout for the field drills is simple by design, but will really get your heart and legs pumping. Follow the chart as you progress through the Boot Camp Workout.

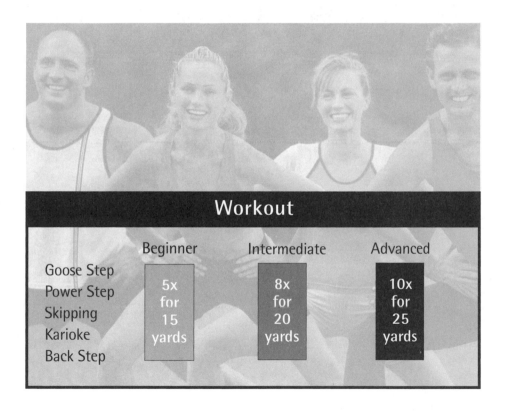

	Beginner	Intermediate	Advanced
Goose Step			
Power Step	5x for 15 yards	8x for 20 yards	10x for 25 yards
Skipping			
Karioke			
Back Step			

BOX DRILLS

Box drills are similar to the field drills, except you will be changing directions in the shape of a four-sided box instead of running in a straight line as with the field drills. The chart below will explain how to set up your box drill course using the same exercises as in the field drills.

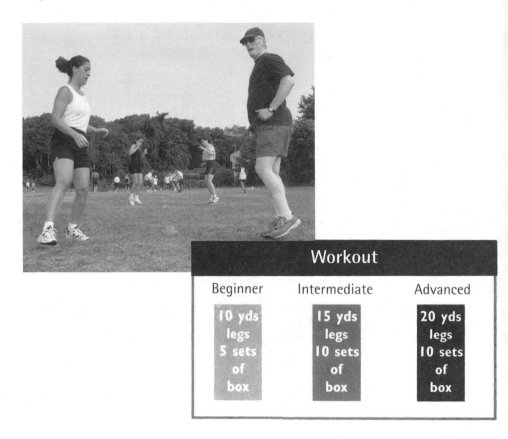

Workout		
Beginner	Intermediate	Advanced
10 yds legs 5 sets of box	15 yds legs 10 sets of box	20 yds legs 10 sets of box

The Box Drill:

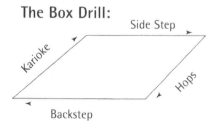

SPRINTS

Follow this workout by running on firm, flat ground (no pot holes) for very short distances. Eventually, as the weeks go by, you will be able to increase the distance and number of times you run these sprints. The object of sprinting is to run as fast as you can.

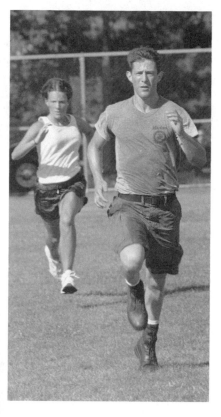

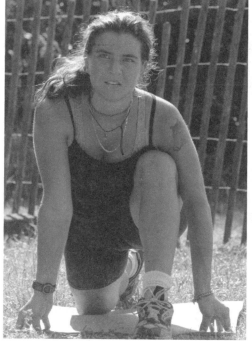

REST DAY / STRETCH

This a day to relax and stretch those tight legs and arms. Now, you do not have to make one day your "day-off." You can move it to any day that is convenient for you. However, you want to exercise FIVE times per week and rest TWO days per week.

UPPER BODY / RUN DAY

The upper body PT pull-ups will be very similar to the regular Pull-Up Workout. There are a few differences. For instance, you are required to do only ONE pull-up FOUR separate times.

If you cannot do a pull-up, remember to give all you have to doing a "negative" pull-up. Fight gravity all the way down until your arms are straight and you are hanging freely from the bar.

Alternating Upper Body PT

This is a quick workout that requires you to move quickly between exercises and sets. Here is what a typical dip/push-up/crunch workout entails.

Set #1 (no rest in between exercises):
    2 bench dips
    3 push-ups
    10 crunches
    Go immediately into the next set.

Set #2 (no rest in between exercises):
    4 bench dips
    6 push-ups
    20 crunches — and so on

The goal of this workout is to build muscle stamina and endurance. This is a great way to perform remarkably high repetitions with relatively minimal effort. This workout is very similar to the superset.

RUNNING TECHNIQUES

This workout is commonly referred to as "interval training." The object is to warm up with a walk or a jog, then sprint for a certain distance as fast as you can. You will not be sprinting during the mild workout, but you will be jogging and walking. Here are a few tips to help you as you pick up the speed to "double time."

1) **Breathing**—Take big, deep inhalations and exhalations. This will help you receive the oxygen your body needs. Too many people breathe too shallowly when they run, causing a hyperventilation effect. Slow down if you need to in order to breathe comfortably.

2) **Stride and Heel-Toe Contact**—Open your stride to a point where you will land on your heels and roll across your foot, pushing off the ground with your toes. Many people run flat-footed or on their toes, causing stress on their lower back, hips, knees and ankles. You can practically eliminate this by following the simple audio test. If you can hear your feet hitting the ground loudly when you run, then you are running incorrectly and may develop tight muscles or painful shin splints. When you're running well, it should sound like your shoes are rolling on the ground.

3) **Arm Swing**—You should have a relaxed, but pronounced, arm swing. Swing your hands from about chest high to just past your hips. The term "hip to lip" is a good way to remember this when you are running. Your arms should be slightly bent but not flexed.

4) **Relaxed Upper body**—You should relax your hands, arms, shoulders, and face. Too many people clench their fists and grit their teeth when they run. This causes the blood and oxygen that you need in your legs to go to your upper body instead. The only things that need to be working when you are running are your lungs and your legs.

LOVE HANDLE EXERCISES

This workout isolates one of man's biggest trouble spots—the LOVE HAN-DLES! Here is Five Star's three phase attack on this menace.

PHASE ONE	PHASE TWO	PHASE THREE
Oblique sit-ups	Butt Wiggles	Side crunches

These are three different exercises that isolate the side of your lower torso differently. Simply read the instructions on how to perform the exercises properly in Part I and do the required number of reps.

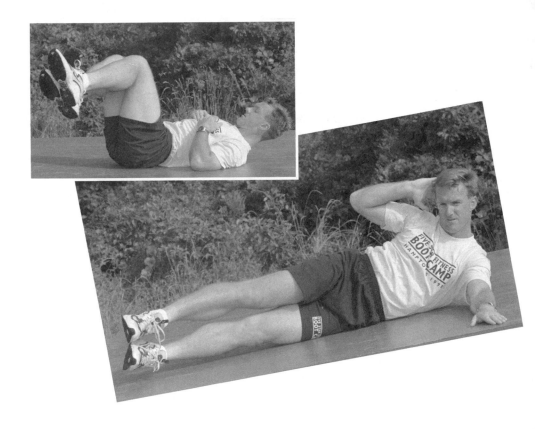

TEST DAY

One day of the week, you will check your progress in two areas: running/walking and upper-body strength. Simply walk or run as fast as you can for the specified distance, stretching your legs afterwards, and then complete the abdominal exercises. Then, test yourself by performing the maximum number of push-ups you can do in a two minute time period. After a two minute rest, do as many pull-ups as you can. Even if you cannot do a single push-up or pull-up, test yourself by seeing how many negatives you can perform for a solid two minutes. Stretch out well before attempting this test. You will be amazed at your progress after a few weeks of practice.

Testing yourself every week gives you a challenge and a goal to reach on a regular basis. Seeing your progress is what makes fitness fun.

So, make some goals for yourself and give it your all to achieve them on TEST DAY. Here is an example of a progress chart you can use to measure your progress.

Progress Chart

EXERCISE	BEGINNER	INTERMEDIATE	ADVANCED
Pull-ups	zero	less than 5	greater than 5
Push-ups	less than 10	greater than 10	greater than 20
Bench Dips	less than 10	greater than 10	greater than 20
Crunches	less than 20	greater than 20	greater than 50
Walk	14:00/mile	12:00/mile	10:00/mile
Run	N/A	9:00/mile	8:00/mile

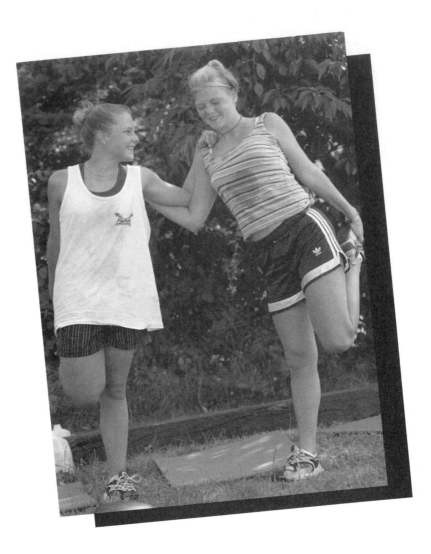

Schedules

Schedules

At the Five Star Fitness Boot Camp, we liked to do things a little differently. One challenge we faced was that each class consisted of men and women at a variety of fitness levels. Beginners, intermediates, and advanced workout warriors were all present. Rather than separate the group or label anyone's fitness abilities, we opted to eliminate the terms beginner, intermediate, and advanced, and introduce the idea of the *salsa workout.*

The *salsa workout* concept is easy to understand. Some people prefer their salsa mild, some medium, and some spicy, and the same holds true for their workouts. At the beginning of each day, through a show of hands, the class would decide how they wanted their workout. Some days would be mild, other days spicy. And for mixed classes, we'd let people know what exercise variations and repetitions met their spice level. For instance, a pull-up can be mild (inclined), medium (assisted), or spicy (no assistance).

The *salsa workout* allowed everyone to participate at their own comfort and challenge levels in the same class. It worked great at Boot Camp, and we're certain it'll work for you. Some days you might want mild, other days . . . you'll turn up the heat!

= mild   = medium   = spicy

If you have any questions about the workouts or schedules, feel free to post them in our website's discussion area at www.getfitnow.com.

MILD WORKOUT—Week 1

MONDAY

1/4 mile walk
Stretch routine

Upper body PT
Pull-ups:
Negatives
Regular grip   1,2,2,1
Reverse grip   1,2,2,1

Push-up/Crunch
Superset
4 cycles of:
Regular push-up   5
Regular crunch   5
Wide push-up   5
Reverse crunch   5
Tricep push-up   5
1/2 situp   5

Bench Dip   1 x 10

Ab Exercises
4-way crunch   10
1/2 situp   10

Walking
1/2 mile walk

TUESDAY

1/4 mile walk
Stretch routine

Lower body PT
No weight PT:
Squat   1 x 10
Lunge   1 x 10
Calf raise   1 x 20

Field Drill
(10:00 boxes)

Sprints
Skip   30m x 1
Hop   30m x 1
20m Sprint   x 1
40m Sprint   x 1
60m Sprint   x 1

Abs—love handles
2 cycles of:
Oblique situp   5
Butt wiggle   15
Side crunch   20
(each side)

WEDNESDAY

Rest day
Stretch

MILD WORKOUT—Week 1

THURSDAY

1/4 mile walk
Stretch routine

Upper body PT
Sets x Reps
Pull-ups:
Negatives
Regular grip 4 x 1
Reverse grip 4 x 1

Alternate each exercise:
Bench dip   1,2,3,2,1
Push-up   2,4,6,4,2
Crunch   5,10,15,10,5

Jogging
1 mile workout
Jog   1/8 mile
Walk   1/8 mile
Jog   1/8 mile
Walk   1/8 mile
Jog   1/8 mile
Walk   1/8 mile
Jog   1/8 mile
Walk   1/8 mile
*Jog = walk fast

FRIDAY

1/4 mile walk
Stretch routine

Lower body PT
Sets x Reps
Squat   1 x 10
Lunge   1 x 10
Calf raise   1 x 15

Box Drills/Sprints
20m   Sprint x 1
40m   Sprint x 1
60m   Sprint x 1

Abs—love handles
2 cycles of:
Oblique situp   15
Butt wiggle   15
Side crunch   20
(each side)

SATURDAY

1/4 mile walk
Stretch routine

Running
1/2 mile walk

Ab Exercises
Do two cycles of:
1/2 situp   15
4-way crunch   15
1/2 situp   15
Stretch   1:00

Test Yourself
Max push-ups _____
Max pull-ups _____

WEEK 1

MILD WORKOUT—Week 2

MONDAY

1/4 mile walk
Stretch routine

Upper body PT
Pull-ups:
Negatives
Regular grip
1,2,3,2,1
Reverse grip
1,2,3,2,1

Push-up/Crunch Superset
4 cycles of:
Regular push-up	6
Regular crunch	6
Wide push-up	6
Reverse crunch	6
Tricep push-up	6
1/2 situp	6

Bench Dip	1 x 10

Ab Exercises
4-way crunch	15
1/2 situp	15
Back Exercises	15

Walking
1/2 mile walk

TUESDAY

1/4 mile walk
Stretch routine

Lower body PT
No weight PT:
Squat	1 x 15
Lunge	1 x 15
Calf Raise	1 x 25

Field Drill
(10:00 boxes)
Sprints
Skip	40m x 1
Hop	40m x 1
20m	Sprint x 2
40m	Sprint x 2
60m	Sprint x 2

Abs—love handles
2 cycles of:
Oblique situp	15
Butt wiggle	15
Side crunch	20

(each side)

WEDNESDAY

Rest day
Stretch

WEEK 2

MILD WORKOUT—Week 2

THURSDAY

1/4 mile walk
Stretch routine

Upper body PT
Sets x Reps
Pull-ups:
Negatives
Regular grip   3 x 2
Reverse grip   3 x 2

Alternate each exercise:
Bench dip   1,2,3,2, 1
Push-up   2,4,6,4,2
Crunch   5,10,15,10,5

Jogging
1 mile workout
Jog   1/8 mile
Walk   1/8 mile
Jog   1/8 mile
Walk   1/8 mile
Jog   1/8 mile
Walk   1/8 mile
Jog   1/8 mile
Walk   1/8 mile
*Jog = walk fast

FRIDAY

1/4 mile walk
Stretch routine

Lower body PT
Sets x Reps
Squat   1 x 15
Lunge   1 x 15
Calf raise   1 x 25

Box Drills/Sprints
20m   Sprint x 1
40m   Sprint x 1
60m   Sprint x 1

Abs—love handles
2 cycles of:
Oblique situp   15
Butt wiggle   15
Side crunch   20
(each side)

Walking
1/2 mile walk

SATURDAY

1/4 mile walk
Stretch routine

Running
1/2 mile walk

Ab Exercises
Do two cycles of:
1/2 situp   15
4 way crunch   15
1/2 situp   15
Stretch   1:00

Test Yourself
Max push-ups_____
Max pull-ups_____

MILD WORKOUT—Week 3

No Running

MONDAY

1/4 mile walk
Stretch routine

Upper body PT
Pull-ups:
Negatives
Regular grip   1,2,3,2,1
Reverse grip   1,2,3,2,1

Push-up/Crunch
Superset
4 cycles of:
Regular push-up   7
Regular crunch   7
Wide push-up   7
Reverse crunch   7
Tricep push-up   7
1/2 situp   7

Bench Dip   2 x 10

Ab Exercises
4-way crunch   15
1/2 situp   15
Back Exercises   15

Walking
1/2 mile walk

TUESDAY

1/4 mile walk
Stretch routine

Lower body PT
No weight PT:
Squat   2 x 20
Lunge   2 x 20
Calf Raise   2 x 20

Walking
1 mile walk

Abs—love handles
2 cycles of:
Oblique situp   15
Butt wiggle   15
Side crunch   20
(each side)

WEDNESDAY

Rest day
Stretch

WEEK 3

MILD WORKOUT—Week 3

No Running

THURSDAY

1/4 mile walk
Stretch routine

Upper body PT
Sets x Reps
Pull-ups:
Negatives
Regular grip   4 x 2
Reverse grip   4 x 2

Alternate each exercise:
Bench dip   2,4,6,4,2
Push-up   3,6,9,6,3
Crunch   5,10,15,20,25

FRIDAY

1/4 mile walk
Stretch routine

Lower body PT
Sets x Reps
Squat   2 x 20
Lunge   2 x 20
Calf raise   2 x 25

Walking
2 mile walk

Abs—love handles
2 cycles of:
Oblique situp   15
Butt wiggle   15
Side crunch   20
(each side)

SATURDAY

1/4 mile walk
Stretch routine

Walking
1 mile walk

Ab Exercises
Do two cycles of:
1/2 situp   20
4 way crunch   20
1/2 situp   20
Stretch   1:00

Test Yourself
Max push-ups_____
Max pull-ups_____

MILD WORKOUT—Week 4

MONDAY

1/4 mile walk
Stretch routine

Upper body PT
Pull-ups:
Negatives
Regular grip 1,2,3,4,3,2,1
Reverse grip 1,2,3,4,3,2,1

Push-up/Crunch
Superset
5 cycles of:
Regular push-up   5
Regular crunch   5
Wide push-up   5
Reverse crunch   5
Tricep push-up   5
1/2 situp   5

Bench Dip
2 x 15

Ab Exercises
2 cycles of:
4-way crunch   15
1/2 situp   15
Back Exercises   15

Walking
1 mile walk

TUESDAY

1/4 mile walk
Stretch routine

Lower body PT
No weight PT:
Squat   2 x 15
Lunge   2 x 15
Calf Raise   2 x 25

Field Drill
(10:00 boxes)
Sprints
Skip   40m x 4
Hop   40m x 4
20m   Sprint x 3
40m   Sprint x 3
60m   Sprint x 2

Abs—love handles
2 cycles of:
Oblique situp   20
Butt wiggle   20
Side crunch   25
(each side)

WEDNESDAY

Rest day
Stretch

WEEK 4

MILD WORKOUT—Week 4

THURSDAY

1/4 mile walk
Stretch routine

Upper body PT
Sets x Reps
Pull-ups:
Negatives
Regular grip   4 x 2
Reverse grip   4 x 2

Alternate each exercise:
Bench dip   2,4,6,4,2
Push-up   3,6,9,6,3
Crunch   5,10,15,20,25

Jogging
1 mile workout
Jog   1/8 mile
Walk   1/8 mile
Jog   1/8 mile
Walk   1/8 mile
Jog   1/8 mile
Walk   1/8 mile
Jog   1/8 mile
Walk   1/8 mile
*Jog = walk fast

FRIDAY

1/4 mile walk
Stretch routine

Lower body PT
Sets x Reps
Squat   2 x 15
Lunge   2 x 15
Calf raise   2 x 25

Box Drills/Sprints
20m   Sprint x 3
40m   Sprint x 3
60m   Sprint x 2

Abs—love handles
2 cycles of:
Oblique situp   20
Butt wiggle   20
Side crunch   25
(each side)

Walking
1 mile walk

SATURDAY

1/4 mile walk
Stretch routine

Running
1 mile jog

Ab Exercises
Do two cycles of:
1/2 situp   25
4 way crunch   5
1/2 situp   25
Stretch   1:00

Test Yourself
Max push-ups_____
Max pull-ups_____

MILD WORKOUT—Week 5

MONDAY

1/4 mile walk
Stretch routine

Upper body PT
Pull-ups:
Negatives
Regular grip 1,2,3,4,3,2,1
Reverse grip 1,2,3,4,3,2,1

Push-up/Crunch
Superset
5 cycles of:
Regular push-up	6
Regular crunch	6
Wide push-up	6
Reverse crunch	6
Tricep push-up	6
1/2 situp	6

Bench Dip	2 x 15

Ab Exercises
Back Exercises	20

Walking
1 mile walk

TUESDAY

1/4 mile walk
Stretch routine

Lower body PT
No weight PT:
Squat	2 x 15
Lunge	2 x 15
Calf Raise	2 x 25

Field Drill
(10:00 boxes)

Sprints	
Skip	40m x 3
Hop	40m x 3
20m	Sprint x 3
40m	Sprint x 3
60m	Sprint x 2

Abs—love handles
2 cycles of:
Oblique situp	5
Butt wiggle	25
Side crunch	40
(each side)	

WEDNESDAY

Rest day
Stretch

MILD WORKOUT—Week 5

THURSDAY
1/4 mile walk
Stretch routine

Upper body PT
Pull-ups:
Negatives
Regular grip   2,4,4,2
Reverse grip   2,4,4,2

Alternate each exercise:
Bench dip   2,4,6,4,2
Push-up   3,6,9,6,3
Crunch   5,10,15,20,25

Jogging
1 mile workout
Jog   1/4 mile
Walk   1/8 mile
Jog   1/4 mile
Walk   1/8 mile
Jog   1/8 mile
Walk   1/8 mile
*Jog = walk fast

FRIDAY
1/4 mile walk
Stretch routine

Lower body PT
Sets x Reps
Squat   2 x 15
Lunge   2 x 15
Calf raise   2 x 25

Box Drills/Sprints
20m   Sprint x 3
40m   Sprint x 3
60m   Sprint x 2

Walking
1 mile walk

Abs—love handles
2 cycles of:
Oblique situp   25
Butt wiggle   25
Side crunch   40
(each side)

SATURDAY
1/4 mile walk
Stretch routine

Running
1 mile jog

Ab Exercises
Do two cycles of:
1/2 situp   30
4 way crunch   30
1/2 situp   30
Stretch   1:00

Test Yourself
Max push-ups_____
Max pull-ups_____

MILD WORKOUT—Week 6

MONDAY
1/4 mile walk
Stretch routine

Upper body PT
Pull-ups:
Negatives
Regular grip   1,2,3,4,5
Reverse grip   5,4,3,2,1

Push-up/Crunch
Superset
5 cycles of:
Regular push-up	7
Regular crunch	7
Wide push-up	7
Reverse crunch	7
Tricep push-up	7
1/2 situp	7

Bench Dip   2 x 15

Ab Exercises
4 way crunch	25
1/2 situp	25
Back Exercises	25

Running
1 mile run/walk

TUESDAY
1/4 mile jog
Stretch routine

Lower body PT
No weight PT:
Squat	3 x 10
Lunge	3 x 10
Calf Raise	3 x 20

Field Drill
(10:00 boxes)
Sprints
Skip	30m x 4
Hop	30m x 4
20m	Sprint x 3
40m	Sprint x 3
60m	Sprint x 2
100m	Sprint x 1

Abs—love handles
2 cycles of:
Oblique situp	25
Butt wiggle	50
Side crunch	50
(each side)	

WEDNESDAY
Rest day
Stretch

MILD WORKOUT—Week 6

THURSDAY

1/4 mile jog
Stretch routine

Upper body PT
Pull-ups:
Negatives
Regular grip   2,4,6
Reverse grip   2,4,6

Alternate each exercise:
Bench dip   3,6,9,6,3
Push-up   5,10,15,10,5
Crunch   10,20,30,40,50

Running
1 mile workout

Jog	1/4 mile
Sprint	1/8 mile
Jog	1/8 mile
Sprint	1/8 mile
Jog	1/8 mile
Sprint	1/8 mile
Jog	1/8 mile

*Jog = walk fast

FRIDAY

1/4 mile walk
Stretch routine

Lower body PT
Sets x Reps

Squat	3 x 10
Lunge	3 x 10
Calf raise	3 x 25

Box Drills/Sprints

20m	Sprint x 3
40m	Sprint x 3
60m	Sprint x 2
100m	Sprint x 1

Abs—love handles
2 cycles of:

Oblique situp	25
Butt wiggle	25
Side crunch	50
(each side)	

SATURDAY

1/4 mile jog
Stretch routine

Running
1 mile run/walk

Ab Exercises
Do two cycles of:

1/2 situp	35
4 way crunch	35
1/2 situp	35
Stretch	1:00

Test Yourself
Max push-ups_____
Max pull-ups_____

MONDAY

1/4 mile jog
Stretch routine

Upper body PT
Pull-ups:
Regular grip   1,3,5,5,3,1
Reverse grip   1,3,5,5,3,1

Push-up/Crunch Superset
6 cycles of:

Regular push-up	6
Regular crunch	6
Wide push-up	6
Reverse crunch	6
Tricep push-up	6
1/2 situp	6

Dumbbell PT

Reverse fly	6
Upright row	6
Shrug	6
Lateral raise	6
Tricep extension	6
Lawnmower	6
Bicep curl	2 x 8
Bench dip	3 x 10

Ab Exercises
2 cycles of:

4-way crunch	20
1/2 situp	20
Butt wiggle	30
Back Exercise #1	
Back Exercise #2	
Stretch	1:00

TUESDAY

1/4 mile jog
Stretch routine

Running
1 mile run/walk

Lower body PT
Dumbbells PT:

Squat	2 x 10
Lunge	2 x 10
Calf Raise	2 x 20

Field Drills
(15:00 boxes)

Sprints	
Skip	30m x 4
Hop	30m x 4
20m	Sprint x 4
40m	Sprint x 4
60m	Sprint x 3

Abs—love handles
2 cycles of:

Oblique situp	30
Butt wiggle	30
Side crunch	60
(30 each side)	

WEDNESDAY
Rest day
Stretch

THURSDAY

1/4 mile jog
Stretch routine

Upper body PT
Pull-ups:
Regular grip
2,4,6,4,2
Reverse grip
2,4,6,4,2

Alternate each exercise
Bench dip
2,4,6,8,8,6
Push-up
3,6,9,12,12,9
Crunch
10,20,30,40,30,20

Dumbbell PT
Reverse fly	6
Upright row	6
Shrug	6
Lateral raise	6
Tricep extension	6
Lawn mower	6
Bicep curl	2 x 8

Running
1.5 mile workout
Jog   1/2 mile

Sprint	1/4 mile
Jog	1/4 mile
Sprint	1/8 mile
Jog	1/8 mile
Sprint	1/8 mile
Jog	1/8 mile

FRIDAY

1/4 mile jog
Stretch routine

Lower body PT
Sets x Reps	
(No Weight)	
Squat	3 x 10
Lunge	3 x 10
Calf raise	3 x 25

Box Drills/Sprints
20m	Sprint x 4
40m	Sprint x 3
60m	Sprint x 2

Abs—love handles
2 cycles of:
Oblique situp	30
Butt wiggle	30
Side crunch	60
(30 each side)	

SATURDAY

1/4 mile jog
Stretch routine

Running
1.5 mile run/walk
Timed _____

Ab Exercises
Do two cycles of:
1/2 situp	25
4 way crunch	25
Butt wiggle	25
Stretch 1:00	

Max push-ups _____
Max pull-ups _____

MEDIUM WORKOUT—Week 2

MONDAY

1/4 mile jog
Stretch routine

Upper body PT
Pull-ups:
Regular grip   1,3,5,5,3,1
Reverse grip   1,3,5,5,3,1

**Push-up/Crunch
Superset**
6 cycles of:
Regular push-up   7
Regular crunch   7
Wide push-up   7
Reverse crunch   7
Tricep push-up   7
1/2 situp   7

Dumbbell PT
Reverse fly   8
Upright row   8
Shrug   8
Lateral raise   8
Tricep extension   8
Bicep curl   2 x 8
Bench dip   3 x 10

Ab Exercises
2 cycles of:
4-way crunch   25
1/2 situp   25
Butt wiggle   30
Back Exercise #1
Back Exercise #2
Stretch   1:00

TUESDAY

1/4 mile jog
Stretch routine

Running
1 mile run/walk

Lower body PT
Dumbbells PT:
Squat   2 x 15
Lunge   2 x 15
Calf Raise   2 x 20

Field Drills
(10:00 boxes)
Sprints
Skip   30m x 5
Hop   30m x 5
20m   Sprint x 4
40m   Sprint x 4
60m   Sprint x 3

Abs—love handles
2 cycles of:
Oblique situp   35
Butt wiggle   35
Side crunch   70
(35 each side)

WEDNESDAY
Rest day
Stretch

MEDIUM WORKOUT–Week 2

THURSDAY

1/4 mile jog
Stretch routine

Upper body PT
Pull-ups:
Regular grip   1,3,5,5,3,1
Reverse grip   1,3,5,5,3,1

Alternate each exercise
Bench dip   3,6,9,9,6,3
Push-up 5,10,15,15,10,5
Crunch
        10,20,30,40,30,20

Dumbbell PT
Reverse fly   8
Upright row   8
Shrug   8
Lateral raise   8
Tricep extension   8
Bicep curl   2 x 8

Running
1.5 mile workout
Jog   1 mile
Sprint   1/4 mile
Jog   1/8 mile
Sprint   1/8 mile

FRIDAY

1/4 mile jog
Stretch routine

Lower body PT
Sets x Reps
(No Weight)
Squat   3 x 10
Lunge   3 x 10
Calf raise   3 x 25

Box Drills/Sprints
20m   Sprint x 4
40m   Sprint x 3
60m   Sprint x 2

Abs–love handles
2 cycles of:
Oblique situp   35
Butt wiggle   35
Side crunch   70
(35 each side)

SATURDAY

1/4 mile jog
Stretch routine

Running
1.5 mile run/walk
Timed _____

Ab Exercises
Do two cycles of:
1/2 situp   25
4-way crunch   25
Butt wiggle   25
Stretch   1:00

Max push-ups _____
Max pull-ups _____

MEDIUM WORKOUT—Week 3

MONDAY

1/4 mile jog
Stretch routine

Upper body PT
Pull-ups:
Regular grip
1,2,3,4,5,6
Reverse grip
6,5,4,3,2,1

Push-up/Crunch Superset
6 cycles of:

Regular push-up	8
Regular crunch	8
Wide push-up	8
Reverse crunch	8
Tricep push-up	8
1/2 situp	8

Dumbbell PT

Reverse fly	10
Upright row	10
Shrug	10
Lateral raise	10
Tricep extension	10
Bicep curl	2 x 10
Bench dip	3 x 12

Ab Exercises
2 cycles of:

4-way crunch	25
1/2 situp	25
Butt wiggle	30
Back Exercise #1	
Back Exercise #2	
Stretch	1:00

TUESDAY

1/4 mile jog
Stretch routine

Running
1 mile run/walk

Lower body PT
Dumbbells PT:

Squat	2 x 15
Lunge	2 x 15
Calf Raise	2 x 20

Field Drills
(10:00 boxes)
Sprints

Skip	30m x 5
Hop	30m x 5
20m	Sprint x 5
40m	Sprint x 4
60m	Sprint x 3

Abs—love handles
2 cycles of:

Oblique situp	40
Butt wiggle	40
Side crunch	80
(40 each side)	

WEDNESDAY

Rest day
Stretch

MEDIUM WORKOUT—Week 3

THURSDAY

1/4 mile jog
Stretch routine

Upper body PT
Pull-ups:
Regular grip 1,2,3,4,5
Reverse grip 5,4,3,2,1

Alternate each exercise
Bench dip   3,6,9,12
Push-up   5,10,15,20
Crunch
               20,30,40,40

Dumbbell PT
Reverse fly   10
Upright row   10
Shrug   10
Lateral raise   10
Tricep extension   10
Bicep curl   2 x 10

Running
1.5 mile workout
Jog   1/2 mile
Sprint   1/4 mile
Jog   1/8 mile
Sprint   1/8 mile
Jog   1/8 mile
Sprint   1/8 mile
Jog   1/8 mile
Sprint   1/8 mile

FRIDAY

1/4 mile jog
Stretch routine

Lower body PT
Sets x Reps
(No Weight)
Squat   4 x 10
Lunge   4 x 10
Calf raise   4 x 25

Box Drills/Sprints
20m   Sprint x 4
40m   Sprint x 4
60m   Sprint x 2

Abs—love handles
2 cycles of:
Oblique situp   40
Butt wiggle   40
Side crunch   80
(40 each side)

SATURDAY

1/4 mile jog
Stretch routine

Running
1.5 mile run/walk
Timed _____

Ab Exercises
Do two cycles of:
1/2 situp   30
4 way crunch   30
Butt wiggle   30
Stretch   1:00

Max push-ups _____
Max pull-ups _____

MEDIUM WORKOUT—Week 4

MONDAY
1/4 mile jog
Stretch routine

Upper body PT
Pull-ups:
Regular grip 1,2,3,4,5,6
Reverse grip 6,5,4,3,2,1

Push-up/Crunch
Superset
7 cycles of:
Regular push-up	8
Regular crunch	8
Wide push-up	8
Reverse crunch	8
Tricep push-up	8
1/2 situp	8

Dumbbell PT
Reverse fly	12
Upright row	12
Shrug	12
Lateral raise	12
Tricep extension	12
Bicep curl	2 x 12
Bench dip	3 x 15

Ab Exercises
2 cycles of:
4-way crunch	25
1/2 situp	25
Butt wiggle	30
Back Exercise #1	
Back Exercise #2	
Stretch 1:00	

TUESDAY
1/4 mile jog
Stretch routine

Running
1 mile run/walk

Lower body PT
Dumbbells PT:
Squat	3 x 10
Lunge	3 x 10
Calf Raise	3 x 20

Field Drills
(10:00 boxes)

Sprints	
Skip	30m x 5
Hop	30m x 5
20m	Sprint x 5
40m	Sprint x 4
60m	Sprint x 3

Abs—love handles
3 cycles of:
Oblique situp	20
Butt wiggle	20
Side crunch	40
(20 each side)	

WEDNESDAY
Rest day
Stretch

MEDIUM WORKOUT–Week 4

THURSDAY

1/4 mile jog
Stretch routine

Upper body PT
Pull-ups:
Regular grip   2,4,6,6,4,2
Reverse grip   2,4,6,6,4,2

Alternate each exercise
Bench dip   3,6,9,12,15
Push-up
        5,10,15,20,15,10,5
Crunch
        10,20,30,40,50

Dumbbell PT
Reverse fly   12
Upright row   12
Shrug   12
Lateral raise   12
Tricep extension   12
Bicep curl   2 x 12

Running
1.5 mile workout
Jog   1/2 mile
Sprint   1/4 mile
Jog   1/4 mile
Sprint   1/8 mile
Jog   1/8 mile
Sprint   1/8 mile
Jog   1/8 mile

FRIDAY

1/4 mile jog
Stretch routine

Lower body PT
Sets x Reps
(No Weight)
Squat   4 x 10
Lunge   4 x 10
Calf raise 4 x 25

Box Drills/Sprints
20m   Sprint x 5
40m   Sprint x 5
60m   Sprint x 4

Abs–love handles
2 cycles of:
Oblique situp   20
Butt wiggle   20
Side crunch   40
(40 each side)

SATURDAY

1/4 mile jog
Stretch routine

Running
2 mile run/walk
Timed _____
Ab Exercises
Do two cycles of:
1/2 situp   30
4-way crunch   30
Butt wiggle   30
Stretch   1:00

Max push-ups _____
Max pull-ups _____

MEDIUM WORKOUT—Week 5

MONDAY

1/4 mile jog
Stretch routine

Upper body PT
Pull-ups:
Regular grip 2,4,6,6,4,2
Reverse grip 2,4,6,6,4,2

Push-up/Crunch
Superset
7 cycles of:
Regular push-up	9
Regular crunch	9
Wide push-up	9
Reverse crunch	9
Tricep push-up	9
1/2 situp	9

Dumbbell PT
Reverse fly	15
Upright row	15
Shrug	15
Lateral raise	15
Tricep extension	15
Bicep curl	3 x 15
Bench dip	4 x 15

Ab Exercises
2 cycles of:
4-way crunch	30
1/2 situp	30
Butt wiggle	40
Back Exercise #1	
Back Exercise #2	
Stretch	1:00

TUESDAY

1/4 mile jog
Stretch routine

Running
1.5 mile run/walk

Lower body PT
Dumbbells PT:
Squat	3 x 10
Lunge	3 x 10
Calf Raise	3 x 20

Field Drills
(10:00 boxes)
Sprints	
Skip	30m x 5
Hop	30m x 5
20m	Sprint x 5
40m	Sprint x 5
60m	Sprint x 3
100m	Sprint x 1

Abs—love handles
3 cycles of:
Oblique situp	20
Butt wiggle	20
Side crunch	40
(20 each side)	

WEDNESDAY
Rest day
Stretch

MEDIUM WORKOUT–Week 5

THURSDAY

1/4 mile jog
Stretch routine

Upper body PT
Pull-ups:
Regular grip 1,2,3,4,5,6
Reverse grip 6,5,4,3,2,1

Alternate each exercise
Bench dip 4,8,12,12,8,4
Push-up 5,10,15,15,10,5
Crunch 10,20,30,40,50

Dumbbell PT
Reverse fly	15
Upright row	15
Shrug	15
Lateral raise	15
Tricep extension	15
Bicep curl	3 x 15

Running
1.5 mile workout
Jog	1/2 mile
Sprint	1/4 mile
Jog	1/4 mile
Sprint	1/8 mile
Jog	1/8 mile
Sprint	1/8 mile
Jog	1/8 mile

FRIDAY

1/4 mile jog
Stretch routine

Lower body PT
Sets x Reps
(No Weight)
Squat	4 x 15
Lunge	4 x 15
Calf raise	4 x 25

Box Drills/Sprints
20m	Sprint x 5
40m	Sprint x 5
60m	Sprint x 4

Abs–love handles
2 cycles of:
Oblique situp	20
Butt wiggle	20
Side crunch	40
(20 each side)	

SATURDAY

1/4 mile jog
Stretch routine

Running
2 mile run/walk
Timed _____

Ab Exercises
Do two cycles of:
1/2 situp	35
4-way crunch	35
Butt wiggle	35
Stretch	1:00

Max push-ups _____
Max pull-ups _____

MEDIUM WORKOUT—Week 6

MONDAY
1/4 mile jog
Stretch routine

Upper body PT
Pull-ups:
Regular grip   2,4,6,8
Reverse grip   8,6,4,2

Push-up/Crunch Superset
7 cycles of:
Regular push-up   10
Regular crunch   10
Wide push-up   10
Reverse crunch   10
Tricep push-up   10
1/2 situp   10

Dumbbell PT
Reverse fly   15
Upright row   15
Shrug   15
Lateral raise   15
Tricep extension   15
Lawn mower   15
Bicep curl   3 x 15
Bench dip   4 x 20

Ab Exercises
2 cycles of:
4-way crunch   35
1/2 situp   35
Butt wiggle   50
Back Exercise #1
Back Exercise #2
Stretch   1:00

TUESDAY
1/4 mile jog
Stretch routine

Running
1.5 mile run/walk

Lower body PT
Dumbbells PT:
Squat   3 x 15
Lunge   3 x 15
Calf Raise   3 x 25

Field Drills
(10:00 boxes)

Sprints
Skip   30m x 5
Hop   30m x 5
20m   Sprint x 5
40m   Sprint x 5
60m   Sprint x 4
100m   Sprint x 3

Abs—love handles
3 cycles of:
Oblique situp   25
Butt wiggle   25
Side crunch   50
(25 each side)

WEDNESDAY
Rest day
Stretch

WEEK 6

MEDIUM WORKOUT—Week 6

THURSDAY

1/4 mile jog
Stretch routine

Upper body PT
Pull-ups:
Regular grip 1,2,3,4,5,6,7
Reverse grip 7,6,5,4,3,2,1

Alternate each exercise
Bench dip
    4,8,12,16,12,8,4
Push-up
    5,10,15,20,15,10,5
Crunch
    10,20,30,40,50,60

Dumbbell PT
Reverse fly	15
Upright row	15
Shrug	15
Lateral raise	15
Tricep extension	15
Lawn mower	15
Bicep curl	3 x 15

Running
1.5 mile workout
Jog	1/2 mile
Sprint	1/4 mile
Jog	1/4 mile
Sprint	1/8 mile
Jog	1/8 mile
Sprint	1/8 mile
Jog	1/8 mile

FRIDAY

1/4 mile jog
Stretch routine

Lower body PT
Sets x Reps (No Weight)	
Squat	4 x 15
Lunge	4 x 15
Calf raise	4 x 25

Box Drills/Sprints
20m	Sprint x 5
40m	Sprint x 5
60m	Sprint x 5
100m	Sprint x 1

Abs—love handles
2 cycles of:
Oblique situp	25
Butt wiggle	25
Side crunch	50
(25 each side)	

SATURDAY

1/4 mile jog
Stretch routine

Running
2 mile run/walk
Timed _____

Ab Exercises
Do two cycles of:
1/2 situp	40
4-way crunch	40
Butt wiggle	40
Stretch	1:00

Max push-ups _____
Max pull-ups _____

SPICY WORKOUT—Week 1

MONDAY

1/4 mile jog
Stretch routine

Upper body PT
Pull-ups:
Regular grip 2,4,6,8,6
Reverse grip 2,4,6,8,6

Push-up/Crunch
Superset
8 cycles of:
Regular push-up	8
Regular crunch	8
Wide push-up	8
Reverse crunch	8
Tricep push-up	8
1/2 situp	8

Dumbbell PT
2 cycles of:
Reverse fly	8
Upright row	8
Shrug	8
Lateral raise	8
Tricep extension	8
Lawn mower	8
Bicep curl	2 x 10
Bench dip	2 x 15

Ab Exercises
Adv crunch	30
1/2 situp	40
Butt wiggle	50
4-way crunch	30
Back Exercise #1	
Back Exercise #2	
Stretch	1:00

TUESDAY

1/4 mile jog
Stretch routine

Running
2 mile run

Dumbbell Leg PT
Squat	3 x 15
Lunge	3 x 15
Calf raise	
3 x 20	

Field Drills
Sprints	
Skip	30m x 5
Hop	30m x 5
20m	Sprint x 5
40m	Sprint x 5
60m	Sprint x 4
80m	Sprint x 3
100m	Sprint x 1

Abs—love handles
3 cycles of:
Oblique situp	30
Butt wiggle	30
Side crunch	30
(15 each side)	

WEDNESDAY
Rest day
Stretch

SPICY WORKOUT—Week 1

THURSDAY
1/4 mile jog
Stretch routine

Upper body PT
Pull-ups:
Regular grip   2,4,6,8,8
Reverse grip   8,8,6,4,2

Alternate each exercise:
Bench dip
5,10,15,20,15,10,5
Push-up
4,8,12,16,16,12,8,4
Crunch
20,30,40,50,40,30,20

Dumbbell PT
2 cycles of:
Reverse fly   8
Upright row   8
Shrug   8
Lateral raise   8
Tricep extension   8
Lawn mower   8

Running
2.0 mile workout
Jog   1 mile
Sprint   1/4 mile
Jog   1/4 mile
Sprint   1/8 mile
Jog   1/8 mile
Sprint   1/8 mile
Jog   1/8 mile

FRIDAY
1/4 mile jog
Stretch routine

Lower body PT
Sets x Reps
Dumbbell Leg PT:
Squats   3 x 20
Lunge   3 x 20
Calf raise   3 x 25

Box Drills/Sprints
10m   Sprint x 10
20m   Sprint x 5
40m   Sprint x4
60m   Sprint x 3
80m   Sprint x 2
100m   Sprint x 1

Abs—love handles
3 cycles of:
Oblique situp   30
Butt wiggle   30
Side crunch   30
(15 each side)

SATURDAY
1/4 mile jog
Stretch routine

Running
2 mile run
Timed _____

Ab Exercises
Two cycles of:
Adv crunch   40
Oblique situp   40
(20 each side)
Butt wiggle   50
Stretch   1:00

Max push-ups _____
Max pull-ups _____

WEEK 1

SPICY WORKOUT—Week 2

MONDAY

1/4 mile jog
Stretch routine

Upper body PT
Pull-ups:
Regular grip 2,4,6,8,8
Reverse grip 8,8,6,4,2

Push-up/Crunch Superset
8 cycles of:

Regular push-up	8
Regular crunch	8
Wide push-up	8
Reverse crunch	8
Tricep push-up	8
1/2 situp	8

Dumbbell PT
2 cycles of:

Reverse fly	8
Upright row	8
Shrug	8
Lateral raise	8
Tricep extension	8
Lawn mower	8
Bicep curl	2 x 10
Bench dip	2 x 15

Ab Exercises

Adv crunch	30
1/2 situp	40
Butt wiggle	50
4-way crunch	30
Back Exercise #1	
Back Exercise #2	
Stretch	1:00

TUESDAY

1/4 mile jog
Stretch routine

Running
2 mile run

Dumbbell Leg PT

Squat	3 x 20
Lunge	3 x 20
Calf raise	3 x 25

Field Drills

Sprints	
Skip	30m x 5
Hop	30m x 5
20m	Sprint x 5
40m	Sprint x 5
60m	Sprint x 4
80m	Sprint x 3
100m	Sprint x 1

Abs—love handles
3 cycles of:

Oblique situp	35
Butt wiggle	40
Side crunch	36

WEDNESDAY

Rest day
Stretch

SPICY WORKOUT—Week 2

THURSDAY

1/4 mile jog
Stretch routine

Upper body PT
Pull-ups:
Regular grip   2,4,6,8,8
Reverse grip   8,8,6,4,2

Alternate each exercise:
Bench dip
        10,15,20,20,15,10
Push-up
        10,15,20,20,15,10
Crunch
        20,30,40,40,30,20

Dumbbell PT
2 cycles of:
Reverse fly   8
Upright row   8
Shrug   8
Lateral raise   8
Tricep extension   8
Lawn mower   8

Running
2.0 mile workout
Jog   1 mile
Sprint   1/4 mile
Jog   1/4 mile
Sprint   1/8 mile
Jog   1/8 mile
Sprint   1/8 mile
Jog   1/8 mile

FRIDAY

1/4 mile jog
Stretch routine

Lower body PT
Sets x Reps
Dumbbell Leg PT:
Squats   3 x 20
Lunge   3 x 20
Calf raise   3 x 25

Box Drills/Sprints
10m   Sprint x 10
20m   Sprint x 5
40m   Sprint x 4
60m   Sprint x 3
80m   Sprint x 2
100m   Sprint x 1

Abs—love handles
3 cycles of:
Oblique situp   35
Butt wiggle   40
Side crunch   36
(15 each side)

SATURDAY

1/4 mile jog
Stretch routine

Running
2 mile run
Timed _____

Ab Exercises
Two cycles of:
1/2 situp   40
Adv crunch   40
Oblique situp   40
(20 each side)
Butt wiggle   50
Stretch   1:00

Max push-ups _____
Max pull-ups _____

SPICY WORKOUT—Week 3

No Running

MONDAY

1/4 mile jog
Stretch routine

Upper body PT
Pull-ups:
Regular grip 2,4,6,8,10
Reverse grip 2,4,6,8,10

Push-up/Crunch Superset
8 cycles of:
Regular push-up	10
Regular crunch	10
Wide push-up	10
Reverse crunch	10
Tricep push-up	10
1/2 situp	10

Dumbbell PT
2 cycles of:
Reverse fly	10
Upright row	10
Shrug	10
Lateral raise	10
Tricep extension	10
Lawn mower	10
Bicep curl	3 x 12
Bench dip	3 x 10

Ab Exercises
Adv crunch	30
1/2 situp	40
Butt wiggle	40
4-way crunch	40
Back Exercise #1	
Back Exercise #2	
Stretch	1:00

TUESDAY

1/4 mile jog
Stretch routine

Dumbbell Leg PT
Squat	4 x 15
Lunge	4 x 15
Calf raise	4 x 20

Abs—love handles
3 cycles of:
Oblique situp	40
Butt wiggle	40
Side crunch	40
(20 each side)	

2 mile walk

WEDNESDAY

Rest day
Stretch

SPICY WORKOUT—Week 3

No Running

THURSDAY	FRIDAY	SATURDAY
1/4 mile jog	1/4 mile jog	1/4 mile jog
Stretch routine	Stretch routine	Stretch routine

THURSDAY

Upper body PT
Pull-ups:
Regular grip
1,2,3,4,5,6,7
Reverse grip
7,6,5,4,3,2,1

Alternate each exercise:
Bench dip
10,20,30,20,10
Push-up
10,20,30,20,10
Crunch 20,40,50,40,20

Dumbbell PT
2 cycles of:
Reverse fly   10
Upright row   10
Shrug   10
Lateral raise   10
Tricep extension   10
Lawn mower   10

2 mile walk

FRIDAY

Lower body PT
Sets x Reps
Dumbbell Leg PT:
Squats   4 x 15
Lunge   4 x 15
Calf raise   4 x 20

Abs—love handles
3 cycles of:
Oblique situp   40
Butt wiggle   40
Side crunch   40
(20 each side)

SATURDAY

Ab Exercises
3 cycles of:
Adv crunch   30
Butt wiggle   50
Stretch   1:00

Max push-ups _____
Max pull-ups _____
2 mile walk

SPICY WORKOUT—Week 4

MONDAY

1/4 mile jog
Stretch routine

Upper body PT
Pull-ups:
Regular grip 2,4,6,8,10,8
Reverse grip 2,4,6,8,10,8

Push-up/Crunch Superset

10 cycles of:

Regular push-up	8
Regular crunch	8
Wide push-up	8
Reverse crunch	8
Tricep push-up	8
1/2 situp	8

Dumbbell PT

2 cycles of:

Reverse fly	10
Upright row	10
Shrug	10
Lateral rais	10
Tricep extension	10
Lawn mower	10
Bicep curl	3 x 12
Bench dip	3 x 15

Ab Exercises

Adv crunch	30
1/2 situp	40
Butt wiggle	40
4-way crunch	40
Back Exercise #1	
Back Exercise #2	
Stretch	1:00

TUESDAY

1/4 mile jog
Stretch routine

Running

3 mile run

Dumbbell Leg PT

Squat	4 x 20
Lunge	4 x 20
Calf raise	4 x 25

Field Drills

Sprints	
Skip	30m x 5
Hop	30m x 5
20m	Sprint x 5
40m	Sprint x 5
60m	Sprint x 5
80m	Sprint x 4
100m	Sprint x 3
220m	Sprint x 1

Abs—love handles

3 cycles of:

Oblique situp	30
Butt wiggle	30
Side crunch	30
(15 each side)	

WEDNESDAY

Rest day
Stretch

WEEK 4

SPICY WORKOUT—Week 4

THURSDAY
1/4 mile jog
Stretch routine

Upper body PT
Pull-ups:
Regular grip
1,2,3,4,5,6,7
Reverse grip
7,6,5,4,3,2,1

Alternate each exercise:
Bench dip
10,20,30,20,10
Push-up
10,20,30,20,10
Crunch

20,40,50,40,20

Dumbbell PT
2 cycles of:
Reverse fly	10
Upright row	10
Shrug	10
Lateral raise	10
Tricep extension	10
Lawn mower	10

Running
2.0 mile workout
Jog	1 mile
Sprint	1/8 mile
Jog	1/8 mile
Sprint	1/8 mile
Jog	1/8 mile
Sprint	1/8 mile
Jog	1/8 mile
Sprint	1/8 mile
Jog	1/8 mile

FRIDAY
1/4 mile jog
Stretch routine

Lower body PT
Sets x Reps
Dumbbell Leg PT:
Squats	4 x 20
Lunge	4 x 20
Calf raise	4 x 25

Box Drills/Sprints
10m	Sprint x 10
20m	Sprint x 5
40m	Sprint x 5
60m	Sprint x 5
80m	Sprint x 4
100m	Sprint x 3
220m	Sprint x 1

Abs—love handles
3 cycles of:
Oblique situp	30
Butt wiggle	30
Side crunch	30
(15 each side)	

SATURDAY
1/4 mile jog
Stretch routine

Running
3 mile run
Timed _____

Ab Exercises
Two cycles of:
1/2 situp	30
Adv crunch	30
Butt wiggle	50
Stretch	
	1:00

Max push-ups _____
Max pull-ups _____

SPICY WORKOUT—Week 5

MONDAY
1/4 mile jog
Stretch routine

Upper body PT
Pull-ups:
Regular grip
2,4,6,8,10,8,6
Reverse grip
2,4,6,8,10,8,6

Push-up/Crunch Superset
10 cycles of:
Regular push-up	9
Regular crunch	9
Wide push-up	9
Reverse crunch	9
Tricep push-up	9
1/2 situp	9

Dumbbell PT
2 cycles of:
Reverse fly	12
Upright row	12
Shrug	12
Lateral raise	12
Tricep extension	12
Lawn mower	10
Bicep curl	3 x 12
Bench dip	4 x 20

Ab Exercises
Adv crunch	40
1/2 situp	40
Butt wiggle	40
4-way crunch	40
Back Exercise #1	
Back Exercise #2	
Stretch	1:00

TUESDAY
1/4 mile jog
Stretch routine

Running
3 mile run

Dumbbell Leg PT
Squat	4 x 25
Lunge	4 x 25
Calf raise	4 x 30

Field Drills
Sprints
Skip	30m x 5
Hop	30m x 5
20m	Sprint x 5
40m	Sprint x 5
60m	Sprint x 5
80m	Sprint x 4
100m	Sprint x 4
220m	Sprint x 2
440m	Sprint x 1

Abs—love handles
4 cycles of:
Oblique situp	40
Butt wiggle	40
Side crunch	40
(20 each side)	

WEDNESDAY
Rest day
Stretch

THURSDAY

1/4 mile jog
Stretch routine

Upper body PT
Pull-ups:
Regular grip
1,2,3,4,5,6,7,8
Reverse grip
8,7,6,5,4,3,2,1

Alternate each exercise:
Bench dip
15,30,30,15
Push-up
20,30,30,20
Crunch
40,60,60,40

Dumbbell PT
2 cycles of:

Reverse fly	12
Upright row	12
Shrug	12
Lateral raise	12
Tricep extension	12
Lawn mower	12
Bicep Curls	3 x 12

Running
2.0 mile workout

Jog	1/2 mile
Sprint	1/4 mile
Jog	1/4 mile
Sprint	1/4 mile
Jog	1/4 mile
Sprint	1/8 mile
Jog	1/8 mile
Sprint	1/8 mile
Jog	1/8 mile

FRIDAY

1/4 mile jog
Stretch routine

Lower body PT
Sets x Reps
Dumbbell Leg PT:

Squats	4 x 25
Lunge	4 x 25
Calf raise	4 x 30

Box Drills/Sprints

10m	Sprint x 10
20m	Sprint x 5
40m	Sprint x 5
60m	Sprint x 5
80m	Sprint x 5
100m	Sprint x 3
220m	Sprint x 2

Abs—love handles
4 cycles of:

Oblique situp	40
Butt wiggle	40
Side crunch	40
(20 each side)	

SATURDAY

1/4 mile jog
Stretch routine

Running
3 mile run
Timed _____

Ab Exercises
Two cycles of:

1/2 situp	35
Adv crunch	40
Butt wiggle	50
Stretch	1:00

Max push-ups _____
Max pull-ups _____

SPICY WORKOUT—Week 6

MONDAY
1/4 mile jog
Stretch routine

Upper body PT
Pull-ups:
Regular grip
2,4,6,8,10,8,6,4,2
Reverse grip
2,4,6,8,10,8,6,4,2

Push-up/Crunch Superset
10 cycles of:

Regular push-up	10
Regular crunch	10
Wide push-up	10
Reverse crunch	10
Tricep push-up	10
1/2 situp	10

Dumbbell PT
2 cycles of:

Reverse fly	15
Upright row	15
Shrug	15
Lateral raise	15
Tricep extension	15
Lawn mower	15
Bicep curl	3 x 15
Bench dip	4 x 25

Ab Exercises

4-way crunch	50
1/2 situp	50
Butt wiggle	50
Back Exercise #1	
Back Exercise #2	
Stretch	1:00

TUESDAY
1/4 mile jog
Stretch routine

Running
3 mile run

Dumbbell Leg PT

Squat	4 x 25
Lunge	4 x 25
Calf raise	4 x 30

Field Drills

Sprints Skip	30m x 5
Hop	30m x 5
20m	Sprint x 5
40m	Sprint x 5
60m	Sprint x 5
80m	Sprint x 4
100m	Sprint x 4
220m	Sprint x 2
440m	Sprint x 1

Abs—love handles
4 cycles of:

Oblique situp	50
Butt wiggle	50
Side crunch	50
(25 each side)	

WEDNESDAY
Rest day
Stretch

WEEK 6

SPICY WORKOUT—Week 6

THURSDAY

1/4 mile jog
Stretch routine

Upper body PT
Pull-ups:

Regular grip	1,2,3,4,
	5,6,7,8,9
Reverse grip	9,8,7,6,
	5,4,3,2,1

Alternate each exercise:

Bench dip	10,15,20,
	20,15,10
Push-up	10,20,30,
	30,20,10
Crunch	30,40,60,
	60,40,30

Dumbbell PT
2 cycles of:

Reverse fly	15
Upright row	15
Shrug	15
Lateral raise	15
Tricep extension	15
Lawn mower	15

Running
2.0 mile workout

Jog	1/2 mile
Sprint	1/4 mile
Jog	1/4 mile
Sprint	1/4 mile
Jog	1/4 mile
Sprint	1/8 mile
Jog	1/8 mile
Sprint	1/8 mile
Jog	1/8 mile

FRIDAY

1/4 mile jog
Stretch routine

Lower body PT
Sets x Reps
Dumbbell Leg PT:

Squats	4 x 25
Lunge	4 x 25
Calf raise	4 x 30

Box Drills/Sprints

10m	Sprint x 10
20m	Sprint x 5
40m	Sprint x 5
60m	Sprint x 5
80m	Sprint x 5
100m	Sprint x 3
220m	Sprint x 2
440m	Sprint x 1

Abs—love handles
4 cycles of:

Oblique situp	50
Butt wiggle	50
Side crunch	50
(25 each side)	

SATURDAY

1/4 mile jog
Stretch routine

Running
3 mile run
Timed _____

Ab Exercises
Two cycles of:

1/2 situp	40
Adv crunch	50
Butt wiggle	50
Stretch	1:00

Max push-ups _____
Max pull-ups _____

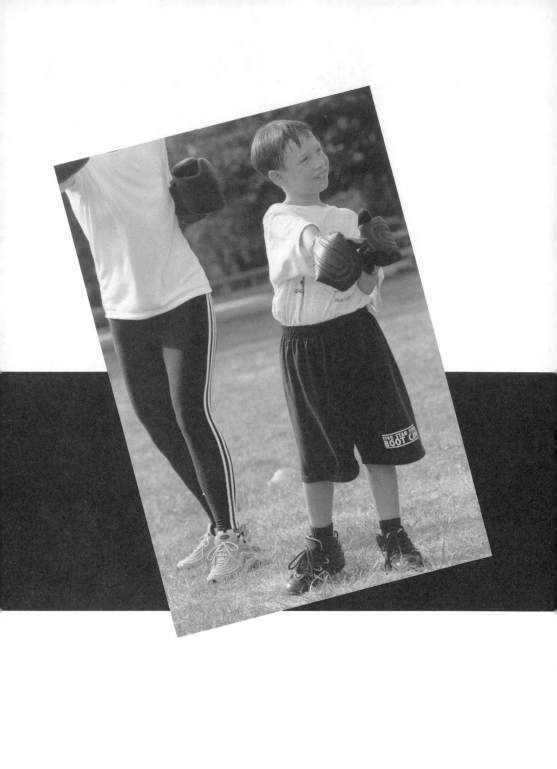

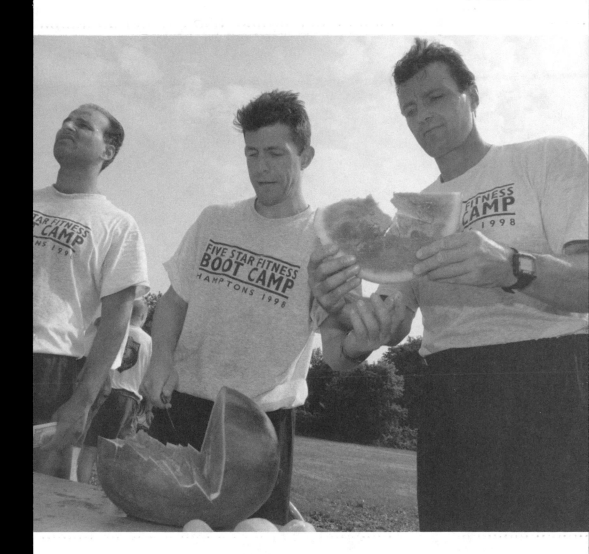

PART IV

Boot Camp Health

Targeting Your Heart Rate

An important aspect to any exercise routine is maintaining your target heart rate for maximum efficiency. During the Boot Camp Workout, we used the Polar Heart Rate Monitors to achieve our individual fitness goals.

An often overlooked muscle, the heart itself is the key to planning a highly efficient, very personal fitness program. Using your heart rate as a guide when exercising can help you workout more effectively.

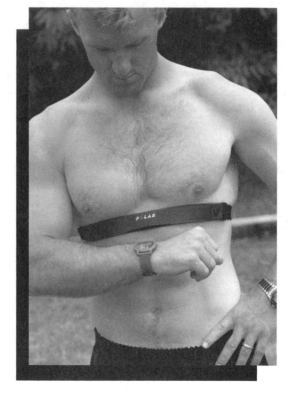

WHY CONDITIONING YOUR HEART IS IMPORTANT

A weak heart is an inefficient one. It cannot pump as much blood as a healthy heart when the muscle contracts. Therefore, it compensates by pumping more often each minute—in effect, prematurely wearing itself out.

With 45 to 50 beats, the heart of a well-conditioned person pumps the same amount of blood in one minute as the average person's heart pumps in 70 to 75 beats. The difference, which is 36,000 beats a day, adds up to 1.3 million beats a year.

Target Exercise Zones

% of Maximum Heart Rate	Exercise Zone
50-60%	Moderate Activity
60-70%	Weight Management
70-80%	Aerobic Training
80-100%	Competitive

UNDERSTANDING TARGET HEART RATE ZONES

When you workout well enough to elevate your heart rate 50% to 100% of its maximum rate, certain improvements in your fitness level are guaranteed to happen. Thus, by understanding what conditioning responses you can achieve by working out at certain levels of effort—known as Target Heart Rate Zones—and by monitoring your heart rate to ensure you reach those levels, you can precisely and efficiently achieve your individual fitness goals.

Whatever your objectives—cardiac rehabilitation, prevention of disease, weight management, or winning athletic competitions—you can achieve them by working out within certain target heart rate zones. These are represented as a percentage of your maximum heart rate, which is the fastest your heart should beat.

For example, if your goal is losing weight, exercising at 60% to 70% of your maximum heart rate is the minimum zone to burn fat calories effectively. To improve your aerobic endurance and really strengthen your heart, you'll need to exercise at 70% to 80% of your maximum heart rate.

TRAINING

You can train within your target heart rate zone only if you know how fast your heart is beating during your workout. A heart rate monitor uses sensitive electrodes encased in a chest band to pick up the heart's electrical impulses. This reading, as beats per minute, is then transmitted wirelessly to a wrist receiver. The monitor continuously tells you when you are in your target heart rate zone.

As you get into better shape, your target heart rate zone will rise. Beginners should slowly build up to the higher part of their target zone. After six months or more of regular exercise, it's okay to hit 75% or, if you are in excellent physical condition, even 80% of your maximum heart rate. The gradual approach is especially important for the elderly, who need longer periods to adapt than younger people. People at high training levels may require a higher training stimulus to continue to improve their cardiorespiratory fitness.

FINDING YOUR HEART RATE WITHOUT A MONITOR

Your resting heart rate can be found by counting your pulse for 60 seconds before rising, when you first wake up. Use the average count of three mornings to determine your resting heart rate. The lower the resting heart rate, the higher the degree of fitness.

During any chosen exercise, your working heart rate can be determined by counting your heart rate for 10 seconds. Multiply that number by 6 to establish your working heart rate.

By pushing yourself to maximum capablitity during any exercise, your maximum heart rate can be measured by taking your heart rate for 10 seconds and then multiplying it by 6. Another way to determine your maximum heart rate is by subtracting your age from 220. For example, if you are 30, your maximum heart rate will be 190 (220-30).

Nutrition and Weight Management

Everyone wants to have more energy to do the things they enjoy. If you want to be energetic, you have to fill your body with the right fuel. Without the right fuel, your body will eventually break down, losing energy and the ability to fight off illness.

This chapter is dedicated to teaching you how to take care of yourself. It will give you basic suggestions and advice on what foods to eat for more energy, how much to eat, and when to eat.

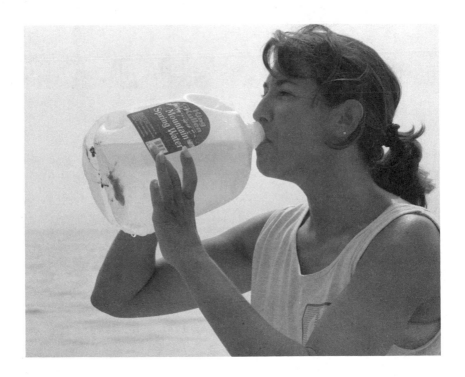

WATER AND DEHYDRATION

Without a doubt, one of the most important parts of your diet is the intake of water. To maintain a healthy and active lifestyle, water is an absolute necessity.

What do we know about the importance of water? You can live for weeks without food, but only for a few days without water. Almost two-thirds of your body is water. Your water percentage must remain that high in order to carry nutrients through the bloodstream to the organs and cells and to remove waste products. Your body uses water every day for breathing, perspiration, and excretion. Although most of us take it for granted, water may be the only true *cure* for permanent weight loss.

According to Donald S. Robertson, MD, MSC, who serves on the staff of the Scottsdale Memorial Hospital and is a frequent source of information for the FDA, water naturally suppresses the appetite and helps the body metabolize stored fat. Studies have shown that a decrease in water intake will cause fat deposits to increase, while an increase in water intake can actually reduce fat deposits.

SOME COMMON FACTS ABOUT DRINKING WATER

- Drinking water is essential to weight loss.

- To get rid of excess water weight, you must drink more water.

- The body can't metabolize stored fat efficiently without being fully hydrated.

- Retained water could be a majority of your excess weight.

- When you drink water, more fat is used as fuel because the liver is free to metabolize stored fat, thus you will lose more weight.

Here is how water helps you lose weight. Your kidneys function best when your body is fully hydrated with water. When your kidneys aren't working at full capacity, some of their work load is dumped onto the liver. One of the liver's

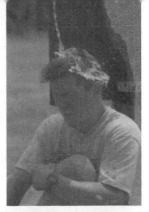

primary functions is to metabolize stored fat into usable energy for your body. But, if the liver has to do some of the kidney's work, it can't operate at full throttle either. As a result, your liver metabolizes less fat, more fat remains stored in your body, and weight loss stops.

Strange as it may seem, drinking enough water is also the best treatment for fluid retention. When the body gets less water, it will resort to what is commonly referred to as "camel mode" and begin to conserve every drop. That conserved water is stored in extra cellular spaces (outside the cells). This shows up as swollen feet, legs, and hands. The best way to overcome the problem of water retention is to give your body what it needs—plenty of water. Only then will the retained water be released.

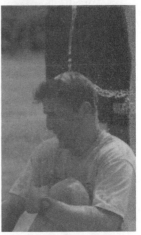

Another cause of problems with water retention arises if you use too much salt on your food. Your body will tolerate sodium only in a certain concentration. The more salt you eat, the more water your system retains to dilute it. Luckily, getting rid of unneeded salt is easy —just drink more water! As water is forced through the kidneys, it takes away excess sodium.

Many people ask me, "How much water should I drink every day?" On the average, a person should drink eight 8 oz. glasses every day. If you exercise and perspire, you need to drink even more water, sometimes as much as ten 8 oz. glasses of water per day. I'd suggest that you have access to water all day and take a sip every few minutes. This will clean your system, give your body its daily requirement, and decrease your hunger at lunch and dinner.

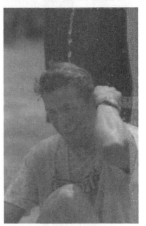

However, the overweight person needs one additional glass of water for every 25 pounds of excess weight. That means, if you are 200 pounds overweight you should drink

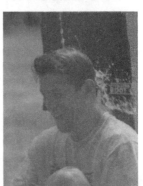

a gallon of water a day. This is because larger people have larger metabolic loads. Since we know that water is the key to fat metabolism, it makes sense that the overweight person needs more water.

Many people think they need to sweat to lose weight. This is not true! In fact, sweating is nothing more than the body cooling itself. The water lost to sweating must be replaced as soon as possible, or you will run the risk of dehydration. Your body can only handle about a four to five percent loss of fluid. Once you reach that level, you will feel sick, tired, and headachy.

The bottomline is that water consumption is extremely important to good health.

Food Guide Pyramid

FOOD GROUP	SERVINGS		
	1,600 Calories	2,200 Calories	2,800 Calories
Breads	6	9	11
Vegetables	3	4	5
Fruits	2	3	4
Dairy products	2	2	2
Meats (ounces)	5	6	7

Source: Modified from the U.S. Department of Agriculture, The Food Guide Pyramid (Home and Garden Bulletin No. 252), Washington, D.C.: USDA, 1992.

FOOD AND YOUR EATING HABITS

You bought this exercise program because you believe you could be leading a healthier lifestyle. To achieve the level of health you desire, the adjustments you need to make are simple: exercise a little more and eat a little less during the evenings and between meals. You should also watch the level of fat in your diet, and avoid foods high in fat. A balanced diet and moderation are two concepts that will help you maintain a healthier lifestyle. It isn't tough to do, if you have clear guidelines to follow.

If you ask people to name the four food groups, many would not be able to answer you confidently. Here is a chart of the four food groups and servings you need per day of each (Fruits and vegetables constitute one food group, but your diet should include servings of each per day).

The chart is based on a 1,600-calorie, 2,200-calorie, and 2,800-calorie diet. Your calorie intake will vary depending on your body type and weight, your age, and the amount of weight you want to lose. Adapt your eating habits to this list and you cannot go wrong.

The biggest change in your diet will involve making breakfast your biggest and most important meal of the day. Breakfast should be your most caloric and nutritious meal of the day. You should follow this saying, "Eat like a king at breakfast, a prince at lunch, and a pauper at dinner."

THE HEALTH RISKS OF A HIGH-FAT DIET

There is a strong association between diet and degenerative diseases such as arteriosclerosis (a high build-up of fat in your arteries). If you eat high levels of saturated fat and cholesterol, such as are found in red meats and dairy products, fat may build up in your arteries. Eventually, the blood flow in your arteries will become restricted or completely blocked, causing a stroke or heart attack. However, certain foods rich in vitamin E (a natural antioxidant) can actually reduce your heart disease risk. These are:

- Fish
- Collard Greens
- Spinach
- Wheat Germ

If you do not like these foods (and many people do not) a multi-vitamin with vitamin E is a good substitute.

A diet high in fats also seems to increase the risk of some cancers, although the exact reasons for this are unknown. Some authorities recommend a diet that allows no more than 20 percent of calories from fat to reduce the risk of breast cancer. *

*Note however, that foods rich in Omega-3 fatty acids, such as fatty fish (tuna, mackeral, salmon), walnuts, and flaxseed oil can actually protect your heart, as well as prevent cancer and other diseases.

FINDING AND PREPARING THE RIGHT FOODS

As with other types of dietary changes, the key word in reducing fat intake is moderation. Drastic changes in your diet are much more difficult to accept and maintain. In fact, a complete change in dietary habits is almost impossible and requires extraordinary discipline. Instead, balance your intake of low-fat foods and high-fat foods. Watch the portion-size of protein-rich foods such as animal and dairy products. Focus on consuming good fats like olive oil, nuts, and omega 3s, and complex rather than simple carbohydrates. Eat more fruits, vegetables, and grains. These foods are healthy, filling, and low in fat, so make them the center of a meal, and use protein-rich foods for accent. So, instead of red meat and cheese, choose chicken or fish and plant pro-

Food Guide Pyramid

FOOD GROUP	SERVING SIZE
Breads	1 slice of bread 1 ounce of ready-to-eat cereal ½ cup of cooked cereal, rice, or pasta
Vegetables	1 cup of raw leafy vegetables ½ cup of other vegetables, cooked or chopped raw ¾ cup of vegetable juice
Fruits	1 medium apple, banana, or orange ½ cup of chopped, cooked, or canned fruit ¾ cup of fruit juice
Dairy products	1 cup of milk or yogurt 1 ½ ounces of natural cheese 2 ounces of process cheese
Meats or fish	2 to 3 ounces of cooked lean meat, poultry, ½ cup of cooked dry beans 1 egg 2 tablespoons of peanut butter

Source: U.S. Department of Agriculture, The Food Guide Pyramid
www.mypyramid.gov

teins, such as pease and beans. Vegetable soup, whole grain bread, and a salad, for instance, makes a great low-fat meal that is loaded with fiber, vitamins, and minerals. Avoid eating trans fats, often found in processed foods and backed goods. These fats increase levels of bad cholesterol in your blood.

Learn how to prepare your foods in a helthier way, too. Avoid frying chicken or fish. Grilling, broiling, and microwaving are good low-fat methods for cooking meats, poultry, and fish.

Let's take a look at the Food Guide Pyramid. Notice that vegetables, fruits, and grains are the foundation of a healthy diet. It is absolutely necessary to eat more of these foods than any other food source. Fortunately,, these foods are inexpensive and an excellent source of vitamins, minerals, and fiber. Vegetables, fruits, and grains are naturally low in fat and sodium and contain no cholesterol. Make sure to eat foods rich in calcium too— from low-fat or fat-free milk/yogurt.

SUGAR

Try to avoid foods high in sugar. These foods tend to have emply calories—calories without other nutrients. Sugar is rapidly digested by the body and provides a quick energy source. If you do not use this quick energy source immediately, your body will store the sugar as fat. Soda is one of the worst offenders when it comes to high-sugar content, and some Americans drink more than twelve cans of soda a day! The sugar in those sodas travels straight to your waist line, buttocks, and hips. Consuming complex starches instead provides a more even, longer-lasting energy source. Eat a variety of fruit, but limit fruit juices—they are too high in sugar.

SALT

Salt, or sodium, can increase blood pressure in susceptible people. Plus, we've already learned that too much sodium can cause weight gain due to water retention. Try to remember that there is really no need to use salt when cooking or eating. Use other herbs and spices to perk up a dish. Many canned and processed foods are high in sodium, so check labels when you're food shopping, and choose fresh food whenever possible. The healthy daily maximum amount of sodium is about 6 grams.

EATING SENSIBLY

Don't feel guilty if you decide to eat a dessert. Remember, "Everything in moderation." If you don't cheat on your workout and diet more than once a week, you'll be fine. Try to cheat only once a week or it will become difficult to lose and keep off those extra pounds.

As you have probably already realized, this entire workout is designed so that you do not have to change your lifestyle or eating habits drastically. Once you decide to make a change in your life, you can accomplish anything you choose to do. So get started exercising, drop a few bad habits, and you'll soon be on your way to a healthy, happy life. Good luck!

Healthy Eating Chart

Food Group	EAT MORE	EAT LESS
Breads	Whole-grain breads; whole-grain and bran cereals; rice; pasta	Refined-flourbreads and cakes; biscuits; croissants; crackers; chips; cookies; pastries; granola
Vegetables	Dark green, leafy vegetables (spinach, collard, endive); yellow-orange vegetables (carrots, sweet potatoes, squash); cabbage; broccoli; cauliflower; Brussels sprouts	Avocados; vegetables prepared in butter, oil, and cream sauces
Fruits	Citrus fruits (oranges, grapefruit); apples; berries; pears	Coconut; fruit pies; pastries

Healthy Eating Chart

Food Group	EAT MORE	EAT LESS
Dairy products	Low-fat or skim milk; low-fat or nonfat yogurt and cheeses (ricotta, farmer, cottage, mozzarella); sherbet; low-fat frozen yogurt	Whole milk; butter; ice milk; yogurt made from whole milk; sweet cream, sour cream, whipped cream, and other creamy toppings (including imitation); ice cream; coffee creamers (including non-dairy); cream cheese; cheese spreads, Brie; Camembert; hard cheeses (Swiss, Cheddar)
Meats	Low-fat chicken or turkey (white meat without skin); fresh or frozen fish; water-packed canned tuna; lean meat trimmed of all fat; cooked dry beans and peas; egg whites and egg substitutes	Beef, veal, lamb, and pork cuts with marbling, untrimmed fat; duck; goose; organ meats; luncheon meats; sausage hot dogs; peanut butter; nuts; seeds; trail mix; tuna packed in oil; egg yolks; whole eggs

Source: Adapted from American College of Obstetricians and Gynecologists, Cholesterol and Your Health (ACOG Patient Education Pamphlet 101), Washington, D.C.: ACOG, 1993.

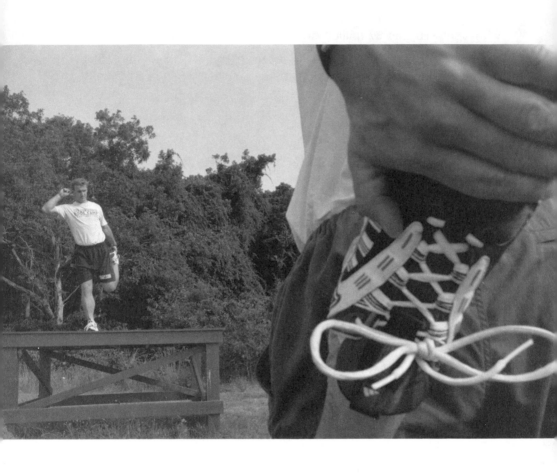

All About Five Star Fitness

There is a growing need for fitness in America today. The National Institute of Health (NIH) recently announced the findings of a study that showed that 97 million Americans are overweight and need to exercise and eat healthier. Ninety-seven million is 40% of the U.S. population!

Five Star Fitness is a new company specializing in the development of products and services for the fitness consumer and fitness professional. Established and funded as a research and development affiliate of The Hatherleigh Company, Ltd., a prominent New York City based publishing and media enterprise, Five Star Fitness is committed to innovation and excellence in all of its endeavors.

THE HATHERLEIGH COMPANY, LTD.

Since 1980, The Hatherleigh Company, Ltd. has developed books, journals, videotapes, and audio tapes for health care professionals and informed consumers. Hatherleigh's products are distributed worldwide.

Aware of the need for high quality information on the subject of fitness for the inactive person, Hatherleigh launched its Five Star Fitness media division in 1997. Initially concentrating on *military style* fitness regimens, Hatherleigh succeeded in capturing the approval of the military branches of the United States Armed Forces to produce a series of *fitness-in-action* books, including *The Official United States Navy SEAL Workout*, *The Official United States Naval Academy Workout*, *The United States Marine Corps Workout*, and

The Official United States Air Force Elite Workout.

Additionally, Hatherleigh is producing a series of books on sports and fitness subjects encompassing a wide range of interests and audiences, such as golf, paintball, lifestyle fitness, and yoga.

MEET THE AUTHORS

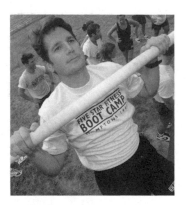

Andrew Flach—A lifelong fitness enthusiast, Andrew is a graduate of St. David's School, The Browning School, and Vassar College. As the President and CEO of The Hatherleigh Company, Ltd. for the past ten years, Andrew's role is directing the research and product development efforts of the Five Star Fitness team.

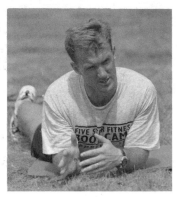

Stewart Smith—A United States Naval Academy graduate and former lieutenant in the Navy SEAL Teams, Stew is a certified personal trainer and author of two fitness books, *The Complete Guide to Navy SEAL Fitness* and *The TV Watcher's Workout.* Stew is responsible for all live training aspects of Five Star Fitness, writing and researching new products, and overseeing the fitness retail and mail order operations.

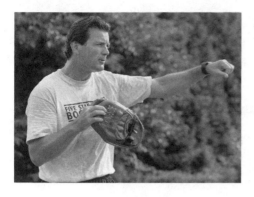

Paul Frediani—An educator for the American Council of Exercise, Paul's interest in fitness began when he was twelve years old, surfing the chilly waters in San Francisco. His interest in sports and fitness lead him to compete in open ocean swims, long distance running, and triathlons. He won the San Francisco Golden Gloves and the Pacific Coast Diamond Belt Light-Heavy Weight Boxing Championships. Paul is certified by the American Exercise College of Sports Medicine and is a medical exercise specialist. He is affiliated with Equinox Gyms in New York City, a Fitness Advisor for Five Star Fitness, and the President of BoxAthletics.

The Official Five Star Fitness Guides

THE OFFICIAL UNITED STATES NAVY SEAL WORKOUT
Andrew Flach, Photography by Peter Field Peck

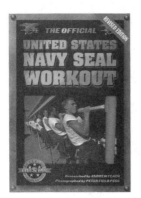

You'll learn what it's like to be a SEAL in this incredible book that brings together the fitness requirements, history, and traditions of the U.S. Navy SEALs. Whether you're seriously into exercising or just want to start a personal fitness program, you can follow this All-American workout to strengthen and tone your entire body.
ISBN: 1-57826-009-4 / $14.95

THE COMPLETE GUIDE TO NAVY SEAL FITNESS
Stewart Smith, Photography by Peter Field Peck

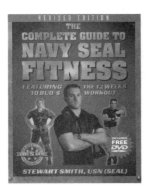

Whether you want to be a Navy SEAL or just be as fit as one . . . here's your chance. Navy SEALs are ordinary people who do extraordinary jobs. It takes an optimal level of fitness to swim 6 miles, run 15 miles and perform over 150 pull-ups, 400 push-ups and 400 sit-ups in one day. More importantly, it takes motivation and determination to stick with it to the end. If you follow and finish this workout, you will find yourself in the best physical shape of your life!
ISBN: 1-57826-014-0 / $14.95

THE UNITED STATES MARINE CORPS WORKOUT
Andrew Flach, Photography by Peter Field Peck

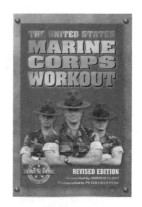

Witness the Leathernecks in action! Come with us as we join Charlie Company at the Officer's Candidate School at the U.S. Marine Corps Base in Quantico, Virginia. You'll discover training techniques you've never seen before. Then you'll travel to Parris Island, South Carolina, where you'll see firsthand the exercises real Marines use to stay in fighting shape. These are rugged workouts for the rugged soul. You want to get fit? Tell it to the Marines!

ISBN: 1-57826-011-6 / $14.95

THE OFFICIAL UNITED STATES AIR FORCE ELITE WORKOUT
Andrew Flach, Photography by Peter Field Peck

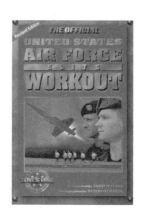

Known as the PJ's and the CCT's, the pararescueman and combat control technicians are the elite forces of the United States Air Force. PJ's, whose motto is "that other may live," routinely put themselves in harm's way to bring back downed pilots and crewmembers. CCT's, "first to fight," are responsible to enter hostile territory ahead of the rest and establish safe landing sites for arriving forces. Now for the first time, their powerful training techniques are brought to light in this profusely illustrated and documented presentation. You've heard of the SEALs . . . now meet their blood brothers.

ISBN: 1-57826-029-9 / $14.95

Available in bookstore everywhere, order toll free at 1-800-528-2550 or online at getfitnow.com.